YOUR HEALTH

An Owner's Manual

Brian Dickens, DO

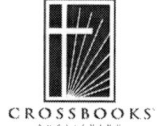

CROSSBOOKS

CrossBooks™
A Division of LifeWay
1663 Liberty Drive
Bloomington, IN 47403
www.crossbooks.com
Phone: 1-866-879-0502

©2011 Brian Dickens, DO. All rights reserved.

No part of this book may be reproduced, stored in a retrieval system, or transmitted by any means without the written permission of the author.

First published by CrossBooks 8/19/2011

ISBN: 978-1-4627-0578-8 (sc)

Library of Congress Control Number: 2011913746

Printed in the United States of America

This book is printed on acid-free paper.

Any people depicted in stock imagery provided by Thinkstock are models, and such images are being used for illustrative purposes only.

Certain stock imagery © Thinkstock.

Because of the dynamic nature of the Internet, any web addresses or links contained in this book may have changed since publication and may no longer be valid. The views expressed in this work are solely those of the author and do not necessarily reflect the views of the publisher, and the publisher hereby disclaims any responsibility for them.

To my Lord and Savior Jesus Christ, to whom I owe everything.

To my loving and supportive wife, Sindy; truly my better half and still my favorite person.

To Steve Dye for his help with photography. If you like his work, you can see more at www.stevedyephoto.com.

To Dr. Matthew Billups, whose friendship and miraculous experience continue to inspire me today.

To Dr. Eddie Dagher, whose insight helped me take better care of my patients.

To proactive patients like Margie McGinley, Dr. Phil Martin, and Linda Martin, who inspired me to write this book.

Introduction

It's your health. Take control of it! You spend fifteen or maybe thirty minutes in the doctor's office for your visit. The rest of the time, you're in charge. How well you do with your health will depend largely upon what you understand about it and what you do about it yourself. Don't get me wrong. Regular follow-ups with your physician are important. My point is that to get the most out of your health, *you* have to take responsibility for it. This means investing the time and energy to learn some basics, being disciplined to use what you've learned effectively, and being proactive with your health in general. This book is designed to empower you to do this.

For the purpose of better understanding this book, it is important to understand a couple of definitions. A DO is a doctor of osteopathy, or osteopathic physician. A DO has all the training an MD has, but also has additional training in musculoskeletal medicine and may perform *osteopathic manipulative therapy* (OMT). OMT consists of a variety of techniques, some of which are also practiced by chiropractors and others by physical therapists. A *somatic dysfunction* is an abnormal position a patient presents in, usually with a limitation of range of motion. For example, a patient who was bent over shoveling snow for thirty minutes and walks into the office hunched over has a flexion somatic dysfunction. His lower back is flexed because extending his back straight causes pain and he has difficulty accomplishing this.

Lifestyle

Exercise

We have all heard the expression "use it or lose it." This is true of our bodies. God designed us to be adaptive. Endurance runners are known to have lower blood pressures and slower resting heart rates, as their bodies adapt to prolonged exercise. Weightlifters are known to have larger muscles and denser bones than the average person.

Unfortunately, when we think of exercise, images of the "no pain, no gain" philosophy often come to mind. In fact, as you begin a workout program, it is likely to feel uncomfortable for you at first. This is because it is a challenge to your body. If it were easy to do, you wouldn't really be doing sufficient work to elicit a change from your body.

My definition of exercise is this: challenging your body in a controlled environment so that your day-to-day activities are less stressful to your body. For this to work, you have to do more during your workout than you do with your daily activities. For someone with a sedentary job, this isn't difficult to imagine. For someone with an active job, however, the mere thought of this can be daunting.

Think of a football player in the NFL. His job is physically demanding. His workout has to be even more so.

For every hour of game time, he has done countless hours of weightlifting, running, and training. Yet his workouts are tailored specifically to his goals.

You may not be an NFL football player, but your exercise should be tailored to your goals as well. If your physician recommends exercise to you, but offers nothing further in the way of specifics, won't you feel a little lost and overwhelmed, not quite knowing where to begin? Your goals may be to lose weight, increase muscle, reduce the risk of heart disease, or even to function better with a mechanically demanding job.

Getting your workout first thing in the morning is ideal for a number of reasons:

1. The first thing you do is the least likely to be ignored.

2. Hard exercise produces endorphins, or "feel-good" hormones. This can lift your mood and energize you for the day.

3. I believe you can get more bang for your buck this way.

Think of it this way: If you've recently eaten something, your body will readily use it for energy. No fat burning necessary. If you've fasted for eight hours (overnight, basically), your body is low on calories and has to scavenge some. Aha! Just why you stored that fat in the first place. It takes about a month to burn fat for energy more efficiently. Until then, you may feel a bit sick so taking a banana or energy drink for a rescue is a good idea at the beginning. Soon, your body gets used to this idea. It's almost as if your body says, "What if he/she does this again tomorrow?" When

Your Health

you do eat, rather than just replenishing fat stores your body will repair and build stronger muscles and bones. Sticking through this first adjustment month is the tough part. Once you get used to it, you'll likely come to enjoy it.

What about those who work twelve hours a day and already have to get up at 4:30a.m.? Then when they get home, the kids want to play with them. Should you really ignore them for the sake of your workout, or get up at 3:30 a.m.? I say no. A better plan is to incorporate them into your workout. Once your child is old enough to sit up without support and enjoy some motion (typically by six months), you can bond with them and get your workout done with the daddy (or mommy) workout plan.

Take some common workout activities: the squat, the bench press, the push up, the overhead press, crunches, and add your child to them. Most young children love to be lifted in the air. Here's a sample routine:

Monday/Wednesday/Friday:

1. Hook your feet under the edge of the couch. Place your child on your lap with his or her back against your knees, which should be bent to around 90 degrees. While supporting your child with your hands, gently curl forward until you're face-to-face. Relax backward and repeat. Do one set of as many as you can. Your child will likely encourage you to keep going.

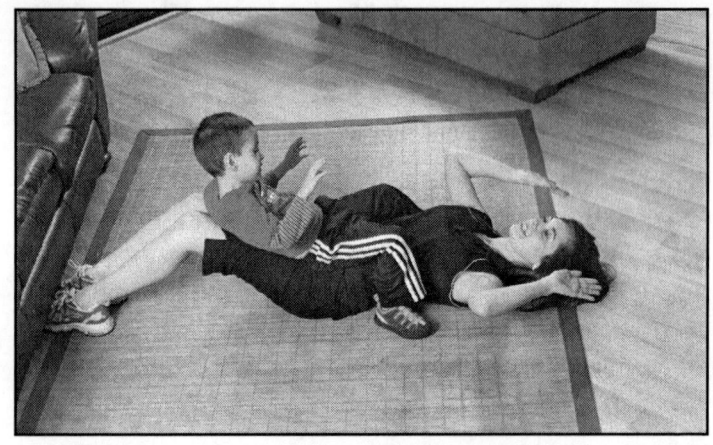

Mommy sit-up

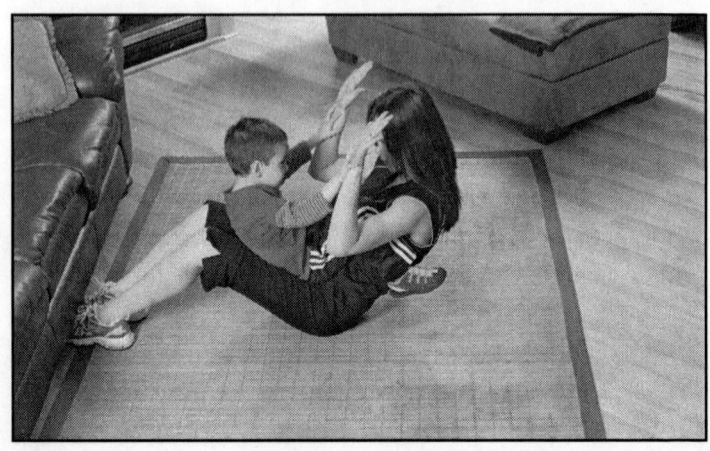

Mommy sit-up

Your Health

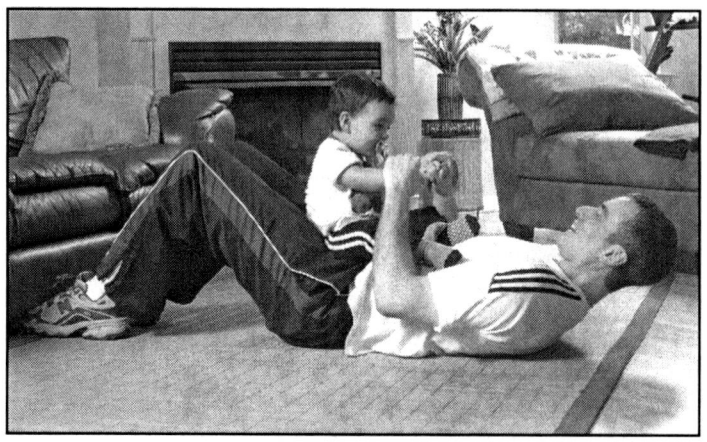

Daddy sit-up

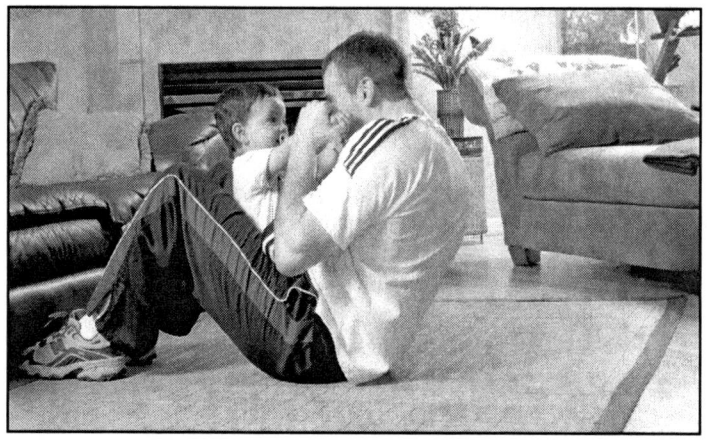

Daddy sit-up

An advanced alternative of this is to lie on your back with your knees bent to 90 degrees. Place your child face down over your shins and while holding his or her hands, pull your knees toward your chest and then extend away. This is a much tougher abdominal workout and requires good balance, so it's not for a beginner. Your child should probably be old enough to walk to incorporate into this one.

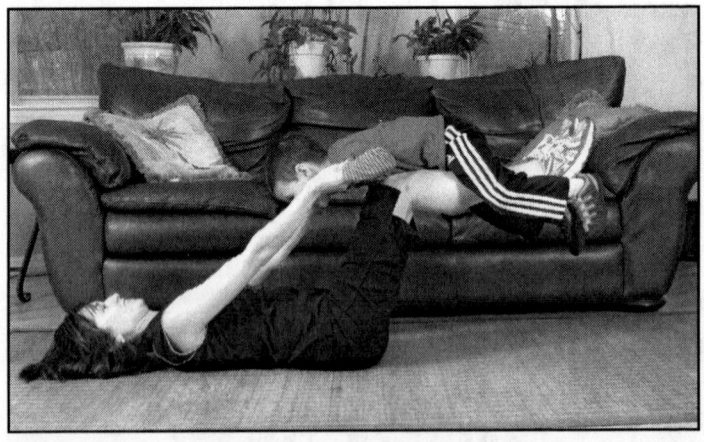

Mommy advanced abs

Your Health

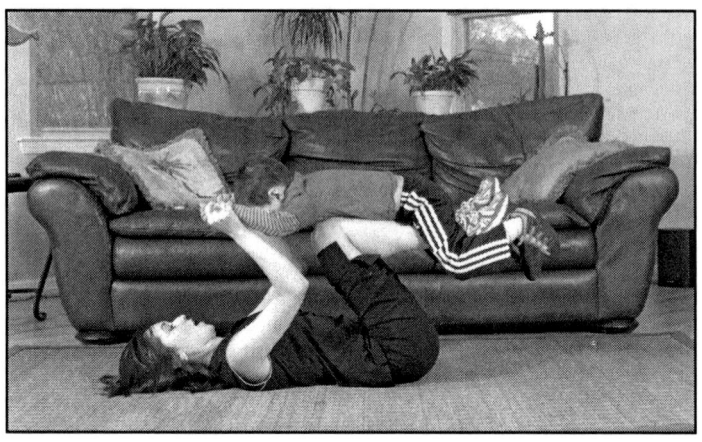

Mommy advanced abs

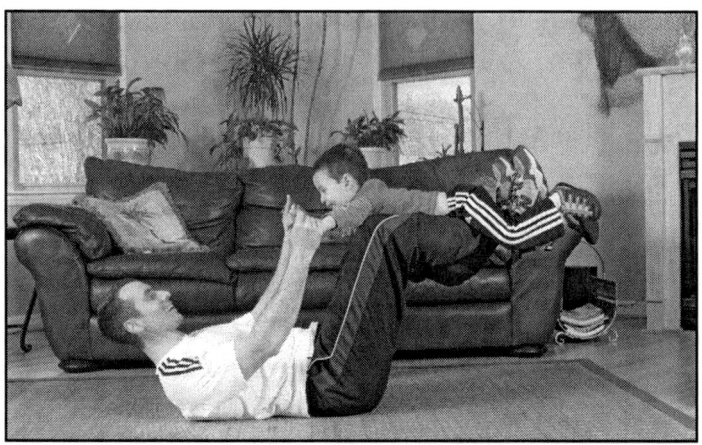

Daddy advanced abs

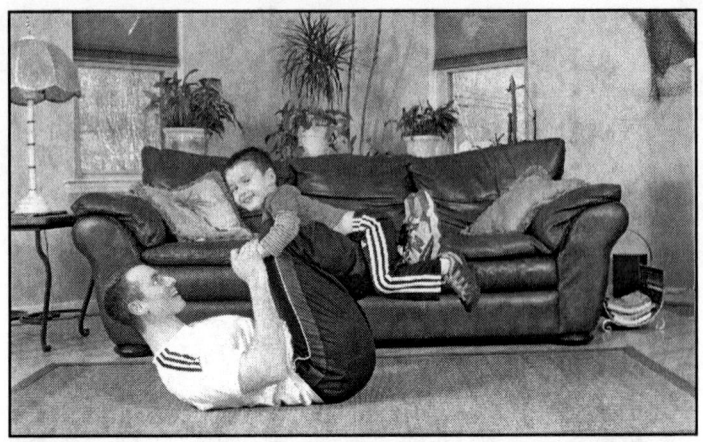

Daddy advanced abs

The exercise with the mother demonstrates isolating the lower abdominal muscles (head flat on the floor). The exercise with the father demonstrates incorporating the upper abdominal muscles as well. Shown with a three-year-old child.

2. Hold your child in front of you with your arms slightly bent. Squat slowly until your butt hits the chair, or as low as you can comfortably go (no lower than 90 degrees). Stand up and at the top of the motion, and lift your child over your head (resist the temptation to toss and catch your child, as this can be dangerous and you still have work to do, anyway). Repeat. Do fifteen repetitions, gradually working your way up to three sets.

Your Health

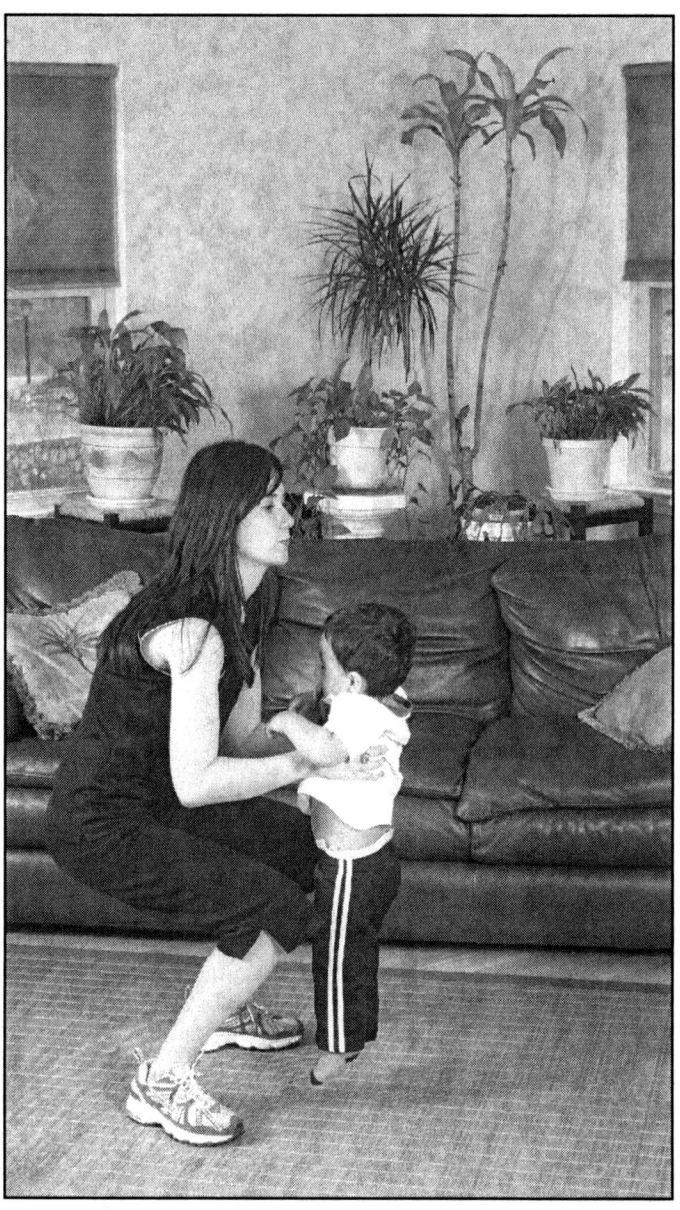

Mommy squat

Brian Dickens, DO

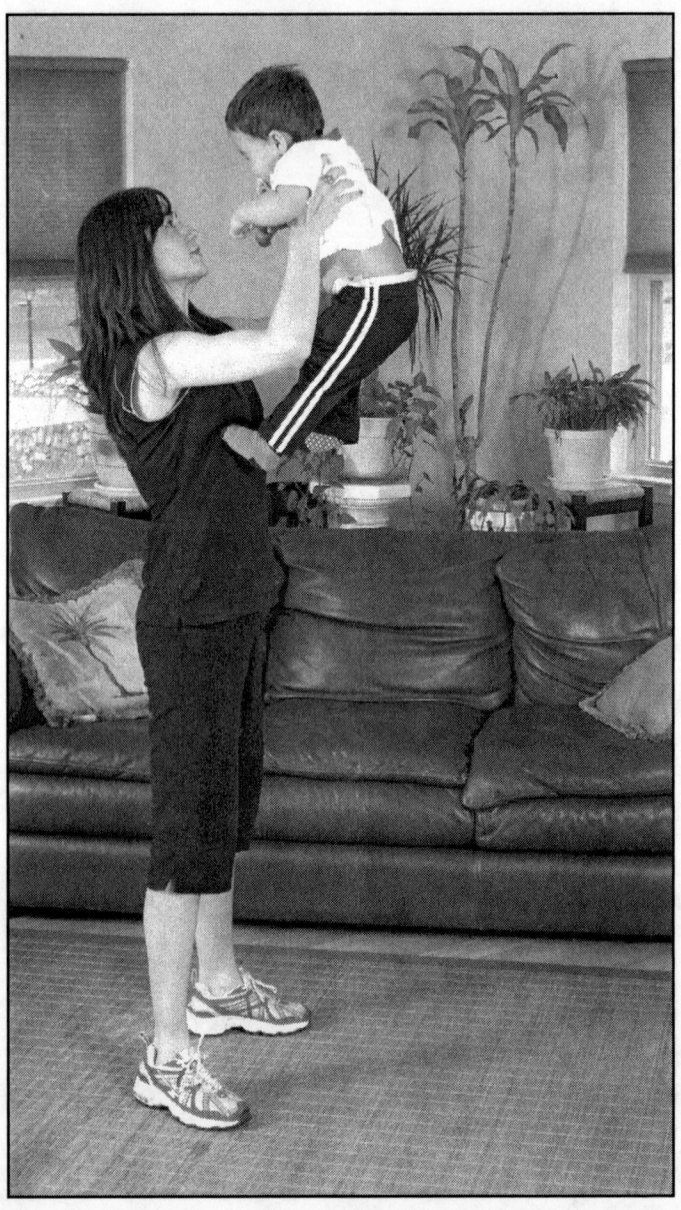

Mommy squat

Your Health

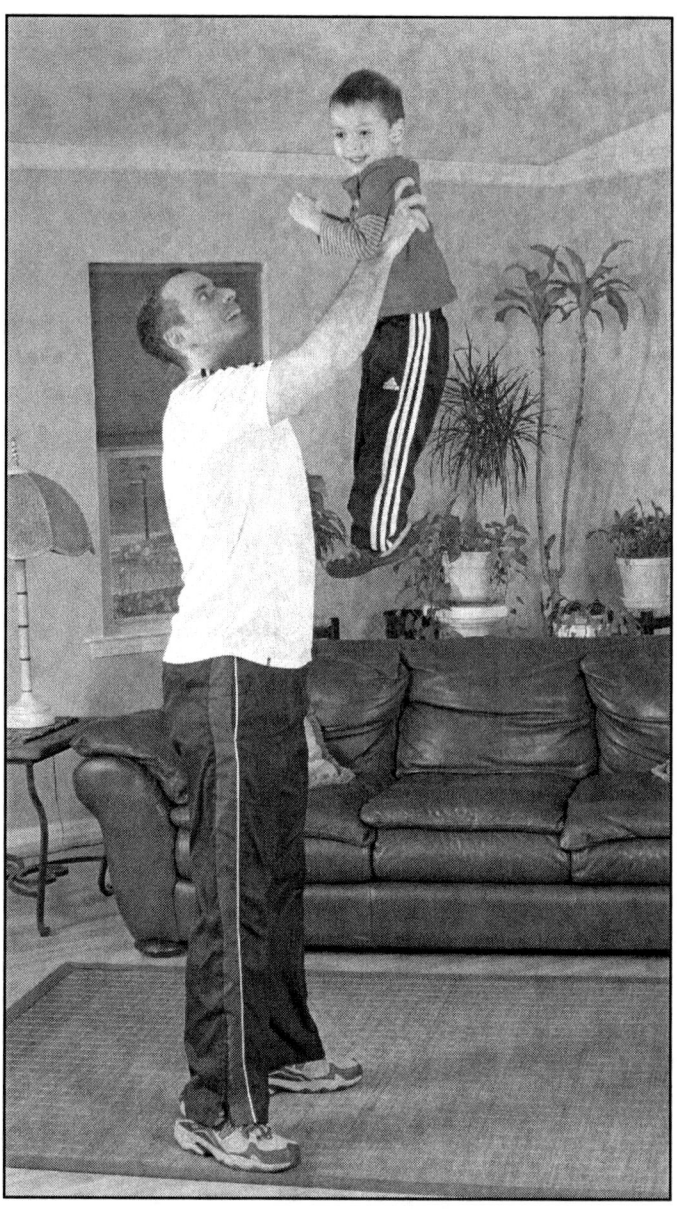

Daddy squat

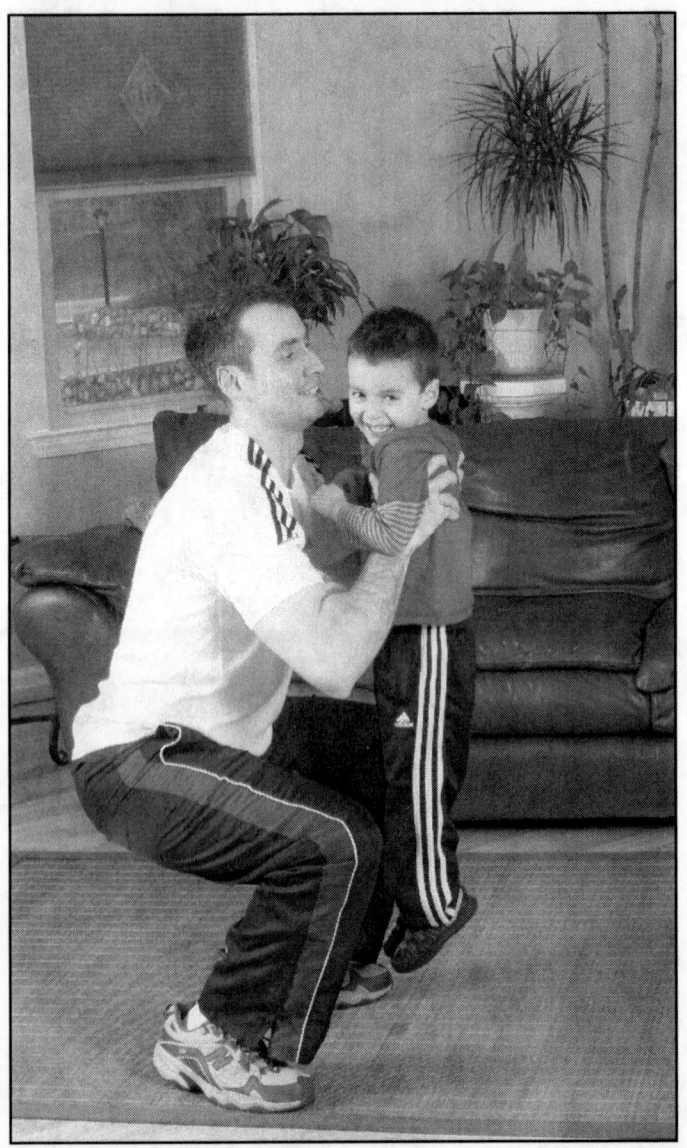

Daddy squat

Shown without chair. May use chair for form.

Your Health

3. Lying on your back, press your child straight up (basically a bench press). Do three sets of ten to fifteen repetitions.

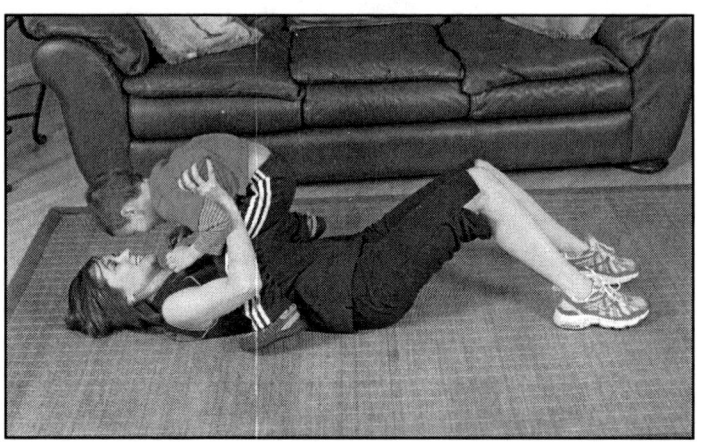

Mommy child press

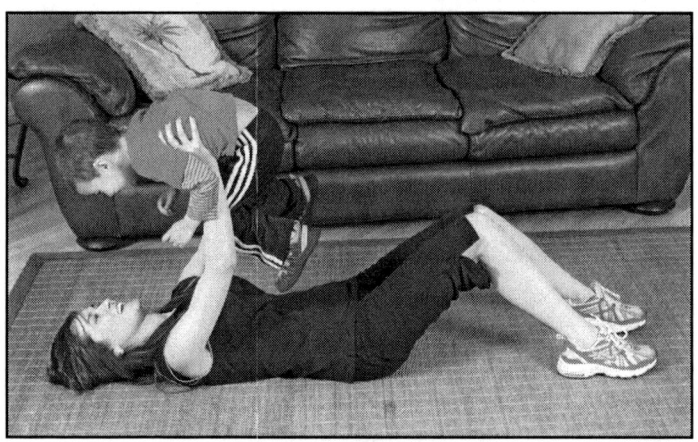

Mommy child press

Brian Dickens, DO

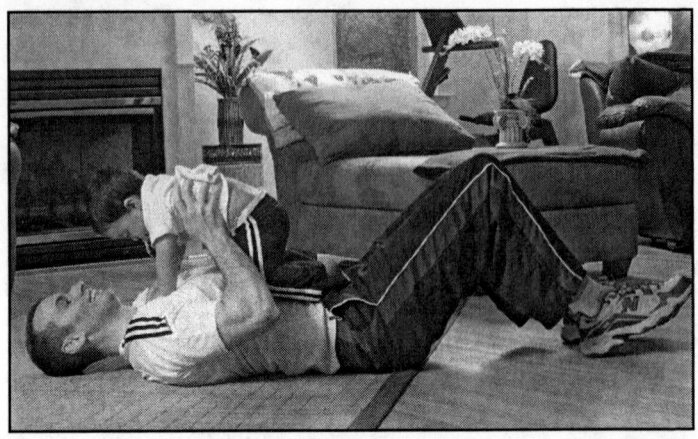

Daddy child press

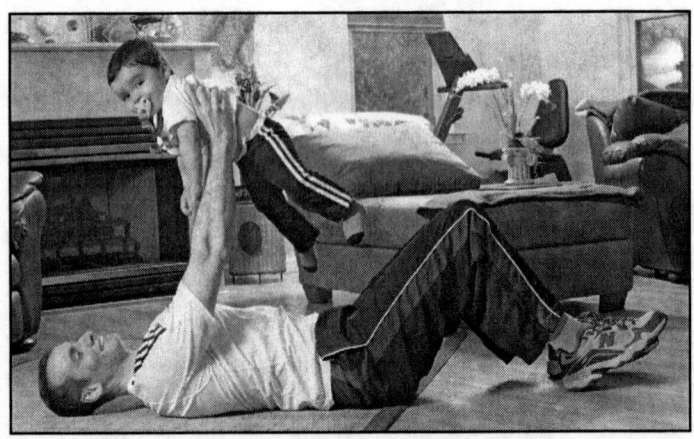

Daddy child press

Once your child is older and can hold onto your back without help, you may have your child sit on your back for added resistance while doing pushups.

It is important to note that before beginning any exercise program, you should consult with your physician.

Your Health

You also need to listen to your body as you challenge it to improve. Chest pain, difficulty breathing, or feeling as if you are about to pass out may be warning signs of a severe, underlying medical illness. If you experience any of these, you should stop your workout and seek help immediately.

Tuesday/Thursday: Cardio day. Walk briskly or jog while pushing your child around the block in a stroller. How far or fast you go will depend on your fitness level and available conditions. A brisk walk pushing a stroller around the mall in the winter is a good activity.

Yes. Technically, this is multi-tasking, but you're accomplishing a lot doing things this way, staying healthy, spending fun time with your children, and equally as important, introducing them to exercise and an active lifestyle.

Exercise may even save your life. I would like to tell you the story of a patient of mine named Margie. She came to me wanting to improve her health. After some baseline questions and a physical examination, she appeared to be healthy enough for an exercise program so we tailored one to fit her goals. Early in her program, she began to experience chest discomfort. The pain quickly subsided when she stopped, but she was prompt to let me know of it.

I recommended she suspend her program until we got to the bottom of her new symptom. I sent her for a stress test, which came back abnormal. Ultimately, she had an 80 percent blockage of an artery in her heart. This was stented, and after cardiac rehab, she was able to resume her exercise program.

Margie had a good outcome. Let's examine why. When you exercise, demand for oxygenated blood to your heart increases. If you have a narrowing of an artery, demand exceeds supply and you get a type of chest pain called *angina*. When you stop exercising, demand decreases, supply can again meet demand, and the pain goes away. Because she was challenging her body in a controlled environment, she was able to tell that something was wrong. Had she actually had a heart attack, there would have been others nearby to help at the gym or she would've been close to a telephone at home.

Suppose she hadn't started exercising. Without challenging her body, she wouldn't have known of the problem. In a sedentary lifestyle, she may have gotten by with only 20 percent of normal blood flow for a while longer. The narrowing of her artery likely would have progressed until she either had chest pain at rest, or suddenly required more oxygen to her heart (maybe from carrying groceries upstairs) that would have caused a heart attack. Being proactive about her health saved Margie's life.

I have had many patients choose to improve their health with exercise regimens. Typically, those getting thirty minutes of exercise three days per week didn't notice much improvement. Those exercising for forty-five minutes five days per week achieved improvement in blood pressure, blood sugar, and cholesterol roughly equivalent to a prescription medication for each.

Most people won't be able to start at forty-five minutes, and if you're new to exercise, I wouldn't recommend it. You could start with as little as five minutes per day and gradually work your way up to your goal. This may sound like a lot, but it actually comes out to only three hours and forty-five minutes per week, or about 2.2 percent of your time. I recommend this as a goal for my patients. You may actually require more, depending on your goals.

For people trying to lose weight, exercise is beneficial whether weight loss is achieved or not. If you compare someone who exercises regularly to someone of the same weight who does not, body composition is likely to be significantly different. Particularly important is visceral fat, or fat around the internal organs. Higher amounts of visceral fat are thought to increase the risk of heart disease. Those who exercise regularly tend to have less fat overall than those who do not, and in particular have a lower percentage of body fat around visceral organs.

A key to sticking to an exercise program is finding activities which you enjoy doing. If you have a treadmill, stair stepper, or stationary bike at home and enjoy a daily television program, you could easily do your workout while watching your television program. Many of my patients who have worked to lose weight have been successful doing this.

In my opinion, of all the exercises you can do, squats give you the most bang for your buck. Mention squats to most people and images of a bodybuilder at the gym grunting and sweating with hundreds of pounds on his back immediately come to mind. That's an extreme, and I'm not trying to turn you into a bodybuilder.

If you can sit in a chair and rise from it, you can, and in fact are, doing squats everyday. There are four major benefits to doing squats:

- As you age, a bad fall can cause a fractured hip or back. Over time, squats increase bone density to both the hip and lower back, reducing risk of fracture from a fall.
- Squats also improve mobility and balance by strengthening the muscles of the thighs, hips,

and back. This reduces the risk of a fall in the first place.
- Squats strengthen some of the larger muscles of your body. These muscles act as a furnace, burning fat even at rest.
- Case studies in men have shown a fourth benefit—a natural increase in testosterone levels. This comes without the side effects of injections for testosterone deficiency, and with the other added benefits to your health mentioned above.

I recently had two male patients in their sixties who had symptomatic testosterone deficiency. Rather than start them on testosterone replacement, I gave them a workout program with squats. Both had significant increases in free and total testosterone levels. In fact, after just six weeks, one had an increase in his free testosterone level of over 70 percent.

Another man in his seventies came to me in a wheelchair, having had multiple falls, once even breaking ribs. When I examined him, I noted atrophy of the muscles of his thighs. After three months of therapy aimed at strengthening his thigh muscles, he was out of his wheelchair, no longer falling, and a lot happier.

To do squats, stand with your feet shoulder width apart. Cross your arms. Slowly lower your butt to your seat, counting up to four seconds. Let your butt touch the seat, but don't put your weight on it. Rise to starting position. Don't go beyond the point where your thighs are parallel to the ground. If you have hip or knee problems that limit your range of motion, simply go as far as you can without causing more pain in your joints. Do one set of fifteen repetitions three days per week for the first week. Increase to two sets three days per week on the second week, and three sets three days per week on the third week. If you feel that this isn't challenging enough for your body, you may add weight in the form of dumbbells in your hands or go to the gym and use the squat rack.

If you have a significant knee, hip, or back problem, consult with your doctor before starting squats. Most people are actually able to do these, even those with arthritis. This exercise takes a common daily movement and training your body to do it better in a controlled environment.

Weight Management

More than 30 percent of Americans are now obese. Salty, fatty, and sweet foods are typically the ones that taste the best to us, because they are the highest yielding sources of the fuel necessary for us to survive. There have been lean times and times of famine throughout human history, and in parts of the world that is no different today. Despite our recent economic difficulties, we are not experiencing a famine in this country.

Most of us, however, are descended from people who have survived a famine or two. During famine times, those able to store up energy in the form of fat when food was available are thought to have been better able to survive times when food was scarce. We've all seen families where everyone is morbidly obese. There's no doubt that genetics do play a role. Add to that the social consequences of obesity where people carrying extra weight are looked at as gluttonous, lazy, or taking more than their share, and it can be a devastating problem.

Of course, the problem is not completely genetic. There is a very large environmental component. Take, for example, the environment in southern West Virginia, which has one of the highest rates of obesity in the country. Coal miners or farmers could conceivably burn 4,000 or even 5,000 calories per day with hard manual labor a century ago. A diet high in calories was necessary for survival. Coal miners and farmers still work hard, but labor in general isn't as physically demanding as it once was, and thus doesn't burn the same amount of calories. The diet persists, however. Now add in fast food and we have a calorie imbalance.

Simple mathematics confirms that if you take in more calories than you burn, you gain weight. Compare the three hours and forty-five minutes of exercise mentioned earlier with a work week in excess of forty hours of hard manual labor. With a sedentary job, you may only burn 1,500 to 2,000 calories per day. You could easily eat that in one meal at a fast food restaurant. Even hitting the target of forty-five minutes five days per week you may not touch the calories you take in with your expenditure. There are many diets available, but one thing none of them can overcome is simple mathematics. If you want to lose weight, you have to burn more calories than you take in.

The biggest hindrance to this is hunger. In extreme cases, bariatric surgery either reduces the size of the stomach to that of a walnut, or places a band around the top of the stomach to limit intake. These may help in squashing the hunger, but they are extreme and not for the majority of overweight or even obese people. In fact, many people can lose weight and keep it off without surgery.

At the center of this issue is the stomach. Why do we

have a stomach in the first place? Well, it does break down food, but it also acts as a storage sack, allowing us to eat intermittently rather than continuously. When we fill the sack, stretch receptors in our stomachs send the signal of fullness to our brains and we stop eating.

If we eat large meals, we stretch this sack out, allowing it to hold more food, but also requiring more filling to have the full sensation and relief from hunger. Add to this high caloric density foods, and especially drinks, and we are set up to overeat.

High glycemic index foods are turned into sugars rapidly by our bodies. Insulin levels rise to help bring this energy into our cells, and then fall again quickly, triggering hunger. Eating these types of foods will leave us hungry soon and contribute to our overeating when we do eat next, probably ingesting more high glycemic index foods and repeating the cycle. High glycemic index foods include sugars, starches, breads, and pastas.

Low glycemic index foods include those with high levels of fiber like fresh fruits and vegetables. They take longer to digest and consequently don't get such a sharp spike or drop in insulin levels, keep you feeling full longer, and lack the highs and lows associated with high glycemic index foods. Proteins and fats also tend to take longer to digest. This explains to an extent the success seen with some fad diets where proteins and fats are eaten to excess at the exclusion of carbohydrates.

Newer evidence suggests that vitamin D does more than just keep our bones healthy. It may play a role in cardiovascular health, mood, pain control, and obesity. Vitamin D is a fat-soluble vitamin. This is interesting because the majority of obese patients I have found have sup-optimal levels of vitamin D. The recommended daily allowances for vitamin D range from 600 to 1,000 International Units, or IUs. We can get vitamin D from a variety of foods, most commonly dairy products, but we also get it from sunlight. Getting just enough sunlight to make our skin blush (not burn) can give us up to 10,000 to 15,000 units of vitamin D.

It's not entirely clear exactly how the body is different with its management of vitamin D in obese people. It could simply be not enough sunlight and dairy, and too much television and soda. It could also be too much vitamin D going into fat storage and not enough left to circulate. It does seem that those trying to lose weight are much more successful once a vitamin D deficiency is corrected, if one exists.

So how do we take all this information and use it to formulate an effective diet? First, don't think of it as a diet. "Diet" implies something temporary. What ends up happening with a diet is that the work is temporary and so are the results. Lifestyle modification is much more effective. You have to change your habits. A "diet" that's too restrictive, time-consuming, or boring is doomed to fail.

Here's a list of things to effectively modify your caloric bottom line:

1. Do the math. Intake and output should be the same to maintain weight. Intake > output = weight gain. Intake < output = weight loss. Period. Many patients vastly underestimate their caloric intake until they see it on paper. If you're putting in good effort to lose weight but are not successful, try keeping a food journal

for a couple of weeks and talk to your doctor about it. Sometimes a metabolic disorder, such as hypothyroidism, may play a role as well, and this is important not to overlook.

2. Know your glycemic index. Low is your goal. Change the habit of your diet to include these foods in place of their higher index counterparts. If you want some juice, eat the fruit instead. In general, whole, less-refined foods are better for you than highly processed or refined foods. I recommend a goal of 30g of fiber daily.

3. Eat more ... frequently. Eating five or even six small meals rather than two or three large ones actually reduces total caloric intake and hunger while increasing energy. Keep in mind that this takes some adjustment. This isn't the same as grazing, where you snack all day. When trying to lose weight, ideally you'll eat what you can fit into one hand. Your stomach won't get stretched out enough for you to feel stuffed, because you won't be. You won't, however, feel like you're starving like you would if you ate nothing at all for long periods of time. Over time you will get used to eating a small amount and stopping until your next meal a few hours later rather than gorging intermittently or grazing all day.

4. Be patient. Weight that comes off quickly tends to return quickly. Additionally, losing more than two pounds per week can create problems with your body. Weight may initially come off more quickly for some people, but averaging

no more than two pounds per week of weight loss is an acceptable goal. Keep in mind that if you did this consistently, that would be one hundred pounds over the course of one year.

This will be effective for many patients, but not everyone. If you have a significant metabolic problem or extreme obesity, bariatric surgery may be an acceptable option for you. Talk to your doctor before initiating any significant changes, particularly if there is concern of underlying medical problems.

Diet and Nutrition

Significant vitamin and mineral deficiencies are rare in this country (with the exception of vitamin D), as people tend to drink soda instead of milk and spend more time indoors. Certainly too much sun exposure can be bad for us, with increased risk of melanoma and other skin cancers, but we actually do need some sunlight, if only for a few minutes each day.

A balanced diet with plenty of fresh fruits and vegetables is ideal. Vitamins may offer some benefit, but most are not regulated with the same scrutiny as prescription drugs, and often there is insufficient evidence as to a clear benefit that they offer. Some, such as vitamin E, have been shown to be largely ineffective in pill form, but beneficial in dietary form.

Nuts are an excellent source of vitamins and minerals. Vitamin E is found in almonds and hazelnuts. Brazil nuts are loaded with selenium, but they should be eaten sparingly, as you could easily get too much of a good thing.

Your Health

As a rule of thumb, eating mixed nuts once or twice a week is a good idea.

Green, leafy vegetables are full of antioxidants, vitamins, and minerals. Those on the blood thinner Warfarin (Coumadin) should be consistent with their intake of these vegetables, as they are sources of vitamin K, which affects blood clotting. Being on Warfarin doesn't necessarily mean you can't eat greens; it just means that you need to be consistent, as variation in vitamin K intake will cause variation in the effect of the Warfarin, and dosage needs will vary.

Fruits are great sources of antioxidants, particularly grapes and berries. In general, the richer the color, the higher the level of antioxidants. Fruits are also a good source of fiber. Fruit juices at the grocery store are often watered down and contain a mixture of water, sugar, and less juice concentrate. If given the option, opt for the whole fruit.

Beans are great sources of fiber, and in many parts of the world are a dietary staple. They're also frequently effective when added to the diet of a toddler who suffers from chronic constipation.

Glucosamine and chondroitin may have a role in arthritis treatment. Some studies seem to indicate a benefit. Others don't. Studies have been consistent in showing that it is considered safe when used as directed.

So are there any superfoods? I'm not sure anything can live up to this title and what it implies, but there are a few foods that, when added to the diet, can have significant benefits to your health. Beans and berries are two of these, as mentioned earlier. Chia is another.

Chia, or *Salvia hispanica* as it is properly known, is a grain that was once a staple of the Aztec diet. It was called "the running food" because just a handful was reported to give energy for an entire day. An analysis of its contents explains why. Each serving contains more omega 3s than salmon, more fiber than flax, and more antioxidants than blueberries. Almost all of the carbohydrate content is in the form of fiber, and almost all of the fat content is in the form of good, fatty acids.

Chia is also pretty taste-neutral. You're not likely to mistake it for tree bark like many high-fiber foods, or suffer from fish breath as you might with taking fish oil supplements. You can add it to yogurt and cereal, or eat it plain, boil it, or cook it in a number of other ways.

I've had many patients on chia, and I've eaten it as well. Some patients have reported an improvement in arthritis symptoms as an added bonus. Some have had an increase in their HDL (good) cholesterol. Some have found it to reduce hunger and improve energy levels. It also seems to have a surprisingly beneficial effect on diabetics, helping them to regulate their blood sugar more easily. Chia has a number of things going for it to which this may be attributable—high fiber, high omega 3 content, and high levels of chromium, which may have additional benefits to diabetics. My own observation is that it seems that patients incorporating chia into their diets seem to have much better glycemic control than those who don't.

Another food that may fit the superfood category is quinoa. Grown in high altitudes like the Andes of Peru and more recently in Colorado, this grain is loaded with protein and other nutrients. It can be used in place of rice in a variety of dishes. I expect to see this become more mainstream in American cuisine along with chia as a growing number of Americans demand healthier options in our diets.

A word about over-the-counter supplements; just because they're over-the-counter doesn't necessarily mean they're safe. They tend to lack the same level of regulation of prescription drugs. A particular problem can be interactions with prescription medications you are taking. Before starting a new supplement, I recommend discussing it with your doctor or pharmacist.

Health Maintenance

An ounce of prevention is worth a pound of cure. Knowing what health maintenance you're due for and getting it is likely to improve your health and may save your life. Immunizations, cancer screenings, and heart disease prevention are key to improving the length and quality of your life.

In the United States, we benefit from a thing called herd immunity. If enough members of a community are immunized against a disease, that disease will rarely be seen and those choosing not to be immunized will still be protected from the disease by virtue of their neighbors who have. That's probably fine if you never leave home.

Keep in mind that infectious disease has killed more people throughout human history than all other causes combined. As a society in whole, we are much better off to immunize than not. Further, traveling internationally may expose you to diseases that you otherwise would not come in contact with. If you travel abroad, contact your local health department or travel clinic and get the recommended immunizations.

Many cancers can be prevented with proper screening. One in eight women will get breast cancer. Catching it early is key to survival. Women with a strong family history of the disease in particular should be sure to get appropriate screening.

Most colon cancers are precancerous polyps before they become cancer. When found early and removed, they never get the chance to become cancer.

Prostate cancer is another story. Most men will get prostate cancer if they live long enough, but the vast majority of these will die from something else. There is at this time insufficient evidence to recommend for or against routine prostate cancer screening in men without a family history of the disease. Those with urinary symptoms or family history of early prostate cancer probably should be screened, however.

One of the most overlooked forms of cancer is skin cancer. Those with fair skin, blue eyes, and lots of sun exposure, particularly as a child or young adult, are at increased risk, but anyone can get the disease. Remember the A–B–C–Ds of melanoma—asymmetry, border, color, and diameter. Any lesion with an asymmetrical or irregular border, a change in color, size, or other signs of change should be brought to your doctor's attention. Non-melanoma skin cancers are more common. In general, if a skin lesion is of concern to you, ask your doctor about it. Don't forget to check the ears. Men who work outdoors are at particular risk of skin cancer on their ears. It's an easy place to miss, both when applying sunscreen and when doing skin checks.

Many people recognize the warning signs of heart disease when it's front and center, but often risk factors leave the patient without symptoms until it is too late. Blood pressure can be dangerously high with no symptoms whatsoever. Cholesterol can be out of control, and diabetes can be developing.

Your Health

It's a lot easier to prevent complications of these diseases than to treat events related to them. Untreated diabetes can lead to heart attack, stroke, blindness, loss of limb, kidney failure, and impotence.

Musculoskeletal

Arthritis

Most of us will get arthritis to some extent at some point in our lives. Most arthritis is mild and responds well to exercise. If there is concern for a more significant case of arthritis, you should see your doctor. The most common arthritis (*osteoarthritis*) is caused by a roughening of the articular surface of the cartilage. Cartilage is *a-neural* (no nerves), so it can bump against other cartilage without pain. It's a great buffer for a joint. Bone, however, particularly the *periosteum,* or lining of the bone, is well-innervated (lots of nerves). When cartilage wears down, bone-on-bone arthritis can be very painful.

There are a number of treatment options for osteoarthritis. Glucosamine and chondroitin, which studies have shown to be safe, are a good first option in terms of medication. I generally advise patients to try it for a month. If it's beneficial, keep using it. If not, don't waste your money on it. Tylenol is another option, but from what I've seen it tends to be less effective than ibuprofen, naproxen, or other non-steroidal anti-inflammatory drugs, or NSAIDs. I recommend Tylenol as second-line, and a NSAID if no contradictions to their use exist.

A corticosteroid injection is often beneficial if oral medications are ineffective. Synthetic synovial fluid like *Synvisc* may have a role as well for those trying to delay a total knee replacement. For severe, degenerative osteoarthritis, however, a joint replacement is sometimes necessary.

The above options are part of the treatment plan, but by no means are they the entire plan. The cornerstone to effectively treating arthritis is exercise. The stronger and more flexible the muscles around a joint, the more pressure is taken off the joint itself. A prime example of this is the knee, particularly when walking downhill.

With every step you take, your upper leg bone, the femur, slams into your lower leg bone, called the tibia, or shin. In a normal joint, cartilage, which is a-neural, absorbs shock from this. When this is worn away, bone slams into bone, which is obviously painful. The primary muscle that cushions this is the *quadricep*. This muscle will start to waste away after just forty-eight hours of non-use. Similarly, it will grow when stimulated to do so by exercise. Hands down, the patients of mine who do the best with arthritis are the ones who consistently do strength training exercises.

Upper back and neck pain

A common complaint for many patients is neck and/or upper back pain. If you have one, you'll typically have the other to some extent. Anything from a motor vehicle accident, to arthritis, to simply sleeping in an awkward position can cause neck and upper back problems. If you have pain or numbness radiating down your arms or weakness of your arm(s), especially after an injury, you should see your doctor to be evaluated, as this may indicate a problem with a nerve.

Your Health

Regardless of the cause of the neck or upper back pain, there is usually a muscular component. The most common muscle involved is the *trapezius.* The trapezius is a diamond-shaped muscle that runs from the base of the skull halfway down the back and out to the shoulders. It functions primarily to pull the shoulders back and straighten the neck and upper back. Patients with trapezius spasms will often show a straightening of the natural curve of the vertebrae of the neck.

Three exercises which I have found beneficial for upper back and neck pain are done as detailed below: 1. With one arm straight, support it under the elbow with your other hand or arm. Gently pull the arm across your chest. Hold for twenty to thirty seconds or until muscle relaxation occurs. Stretch both sides equally. 2. With your back resting against the back of a chair, interlock your fingers and place them behind the back of your neck. Let your arms fall forward and gently stretch your neck and upper back. 3. Sitting upright, take one hand and reach across the top of your head, grasping the other side. Gently pull your head to one side, while grasping the edge of your chair with the other hand. You may allow your shoulder on the side being stretched to elevate a bit at the end to get a good stretch of your upper back muscles. Do these stretches at least twice daily (morning and evening), and again if you notice tightening of your muscles.

Other muscles commonly involved in neck pain include the *scalenes, sternocleido-mastoid,* and the muscles of the *suboccipital triangle,* the area where the skull attaches to the neck. These muscles are involved in some of the fine movements of the head. The key to managing neck and upper back pain is to first get the range of motion back to normal or as close as possible. OMT, chiropractic, physical therapy, massage therapy, and acupuncture all have something to offer in treating neck and back pain, and the sooner they are incorporated into care, the better the outcome in general.

The most effective technique for a limited range of motion is, in my opinion, muscle energy technique. This technique is most often used in OMT done by an osteopathic physician, but can also be done by a chiropractor or massage therapist who is trained in it. It involves taking the affected muscle to the limited barrier and having the patient press in the opposite direction for three to five seconds. The patient then relaxes, and via stimulation of a reflex thought to prevent tearing of muscle or tendon, a muscle relaxation is achieved and the range of motion restored. This is done incrementally until maximum improvement is attained. It is important to have this done by a professional who is proficient in this technique.

Lower back pain

Low back pain is one of the more common problems seen in the primary care setting. It is important to differentiate between pain resulting from a musculoskeletal problem versus pain caused by something else like a urinary tract or bowel problem. Presence of blood in the urine, pain radiating down one or both legs, or pain with associated numbness, tingling, or other neurological symptoms should require medical attention.

Most low back pain is mechanical in nature, resulting from prolonged work in an awkward position, working beyond the physical conditioning of your back, or lifting a load improperly. In addition to the benefits mentioned earlier, strength training has the added benefit of teaching proper lifting technique.

Pain considered to be low back in origin is often just a bit lower. A somatic dysfunction of the *sacrum,* which lies just beneath the lumbar spine, or the pelvis, is common and if found early, can often be remedied by OMT or chiropractic care. I have found muscle energy technique particularly useful for problems of the sacrum and pelvis. A problem with the *piriformis* muscle is often associated with a somatic dysfunction of the sacrum or pelvis and may contribute to *sciatica,* pain resulting from pressure on the sciatic nerve.

Another culprit in low back pain is commonly the *iliopsoas* muscle. This muscle functions to flex the hip and pull the knee upward. Dysfunction of this muscle can cause significant low back pain. It is usually affected when the patient has been in a bent over position for a prolonged time.

OMT, chiropractic care, physical therapy, massage therapy, and acupuncture are all beneficial in treating low back pain. The cornerstone for ultimately achieving success and preventing recurrence, however, is actually strength training. This involves the hips, low back, and abdominal muscles, including obliques. Studies suggest that four days of exercise per week for this yields superior results to fewer days of exercise, and may offer approximately 30 percent pain relief. Excess abdominal fat can also worsen low back pain. Losing this abdominal fat may significantly reduce pain and improve symptoms.

Rotator cuff and shoulder problems

The rotator cuff consists of four muscles. The most commonly injured of these muscles is the *supraspinatus.* The supraspinatus runs along the upper edge of the shoulder blade. Tendons attach muscles to bone, and the supraspinatus tendon runs underneath the joint where the shoulder blade and collar bone meet (the AC or *acromioclavicular* joint).

Raising the arm away from the body or across the body will usually make the pain worse with a supraspinatus injury. An easy and less painful test for supraspinatus tendonitis consists of trying to kiss the inside of your elbow. If doing this elicits pain and you have difficulty reaching your elbow, you likely have supraspinatus tendonitis. It is important to see your doctor if you have significant shoulder pain to rule out a rotator cuff tear or other more serious condition.

Treatment of rotator cuff tendonitis consists of a trial of a NSAID (non-steroidal anti-inflammatory drug) like ibuprofen. Your doctor may give you a prescription for a higher dose than you would typically take over the counter. Taking this scheduled for one week will often reduce inflammation enough to allow you to return to normal function. If this is ineffective, a *corticosteroid* injection into your shoulder may offer benefit. The likely reason this is effective is the decrease in inflammation, causing a decrease in impingement of the AC joint on the supraspinatus tendon.

Rotator cuff muscles are small, but critical to stability of the shoulder. In allowing a wide range of motion, the shoulder sacrifices stability, putting more onus on the muscles of the shoulder to stabilize it. Trying to strengthen the supraspinatus muscle while it is being impinged can prove difficult, if not impossible.

A simple solution is turning the thumb upward rather than to the front while exercising. This rotates the insertion of the tendon backward, freeing it from impingement from the AC joint. Simply take a pair of dumbbells or a can of beans at home and raise them to your sides until your hands are at shoulder level. Make sure your thumb is facing upward. Slowly lower over four seconds. Do fifteen repetitions for one or two sets four days per week.

Carpal tunnel syndrome

Carpal tunnel syndrome (CTS) is impingement of the median nerve causing tingling, numbness, pain, and weakness of the hand. People with wrists that are as thick as they are wide are at increased risk of carpal tunnel syndrome. Women are at greater risk of CTS than men. Diabetics are also at increased risk. In severe cases, surgery may be necessary, but often it is not.

First, let's consider the anatomy of carpal tunnel to see why this happens. There is a limited space through which the median nerve and a bunch of tendons must pass through the arm. Tendonitis, or inflammation of these tendons, reduces space in the carpal tunnel, compresses the median nerve, and causes symptoms of CTS. Often, treating this tendonitis will reduce symptoms and allow patients to avoid surgery.

One of the mainstays of treatment is the splint. Be cautious, as this can actually make CTS worse. Pressure in the carpal tunnel is significantly increased when the wrist is bent in one direction or another beyond fifteen degrees. If you use a splint, make sure the wrist is in a neutral position in the splint. If it isn't, you may be worsening the problem rather than helping it.

Finally, if tendonitis is causing your symptoms, you need to treat the tendonitis. This involves improving flexibility and strength of the wrist flexor muscles and reducing inflammation of flexor tendons going through the carpal tunnel.

Tendonitis

Conventional treatment of tendonitis with rest, ice, heat, and splinting has been hit or miss at best in effectiveness. More recent studies have shown that eccentric phase strength training is much more effective. Taking a light to moderate amount of weight, raising it normally, and lowering it slowly over four seconds has shown promise. Do twelve to fifteen repetitions for one or two sets four days per week. If a significant tendon problem is a possibility, you should see your doctor to be sure it is tendonitis you're dealing with and not something more serious.

Fibromyalgia

Fibromyalgia is somewhat of a diagnosis of exclusion. There has been a lot of disagreement as to whether or not it even existed in the recent past, much less in how to effectively treat it. For whatever reason, it appears to be a hypersensitivity to pain. The most important aspect of treatment is exercise. Regardless of whatever else patients do in treatment, it is likely to be ineffective if regular exercise is not maintained. Strength training is beneficial, but aerobic exercise is thought to be more effective in fibromyalgia.

Medications showing some promise include muscle relaxers, antidepressants, and some anti-seizure medications. Narcotic use has not been shown to be effective at treating fibromyalgia and often worsens the condition.

Foot pain

A number of factors can contribute to foot pain. Excess weight, inactivity, and poor footwear are at the top of the list. As a rule of thumb, shoes worn frequently should be replaced at least yearly if possible. If you're on your feet all day, especially on a hard surface, I recommend shoe inserts such as Superfeet. I personally use these and found them to be key in reducing not only foot pain, but back pain as well after long days at work.

Probably the most common cause of foot pain I see is *plantar fasciitis*. Fascia is your body's connective tissue, and your plantar fascia is on the bottom of your feet and runs from your heel to your forefoot. Patients with plantar fasciitis typically complain of pain under the heel or just in front of it, which is worse in the morning or with their first steps after sitting for a prolonged period of time.

The pain associated with plantar fasciitis is thought to be due to contraction of the plantar fascia with rest. When weight is added to it, this fascia is ripped open again as it stretches out. Treatment includes loss of excessive weight, stretching and strengthening of calf muscles and arches, and a Strassburg sock. The Strassburg sock has a strap at the top that hooks onto an attachment near the knee. It holds the foot in dorsiflexion, which stretches the plantar fascia during sleep. Comparable boots that hold the foot in similar position tend to be poorly tolerated, but the Strassburg sock may reach success rates in excess of 90 percent for plantar fasciitis. I recommend it as part of first-line treatment.

Gout

Gout is a condition affecting joints caused by either too much uric acid production or insufficient uric acid excretion. The majority of cases are caused by insufficient excretion, but it is most commonly prevented by taking a medication that lowers production, as this works for either cause. Uric acid is eliminated by the kidneys, and occasionally excess uric acid in the urine can contribute to uric acid kidney stones.

While medications that prevent production of uric acid (*xanthine oxidase* inhibitors like *allopurinol*) are good at preventing a case of gout, they can actually exacerbate a current flare. To treat an acute attack, a non-steroidal anti-inflammatory like Indomethicin is ideal.

These medications can be hard on your kidneys, however, and if this is the case, an anti-inflammatory such as Prednisone is usually prescribed. Prednisone can raise blood sugars, however, and many gout-sufferers also have—you guessed it—diabetes.

In this case, colchicine can be used. This medication, while effective, has a nasty little side effect of diarrhea, which may render you socially unavailable. In this case, it may be necessary to go with the Prednisone, realizing that blood sugars will temporarily run high and likely cause an increase in insulin for insulin-dependent diabetics until the course of treatment is completed.

Narcotic use in pain management

Narcotics treat pain by mimicking a reaction our bodies naturally produce in response to severe pain. With chronic use of narcotics, your brain gets the message "Hey! I can't feel anything," and adjusts to allow you to feel again. Higher doses become necessary to achieve the same pain reduction over time. After three to four months of taking narcotics, many patients actually function worse and have more pain than patients with the same condition who are not on narcotics. I've actually had a number of patients who experienced less pain when exercise was added and narcotics were removed.

Narcotic use in chronic, non-malignant pain often does more harm than good. In addition to the well-known risks of dependence and addiction, narcotics may cause constipation and actually worsen pain. They can also cause problems with your endocrine system, your thyroid, adrenals, and sex hormones. In fact, chronic use of narcotics can significantly suppress testosterone production in men.

Mental Health

Smoking

If you're a smoker, I recommend you stop, and it won't be easy. Most smokers try and fail in cessation attempts many times before finally succeeding. Approximately 5 percent of patients will quit smoking and maintain smoke free lifestyles if their physician recommends it. 20 percent or more will successfully quit if they have an organized plan and are counseled on this. Smoking is a medical problem just like diabetes or hypertension, and to be treated successfully, it needs to be treated as such.

Smoking affects not only your lungs, but it also affects your cardiovascular system. Several studies have shown a reduction in hospital admissions for heart attacks after smoking was banned in public places. Not only should you refrain from smoking, or stop altogether if you do smoke, you also shouldn't let anyone smoke around you or your loved ones.

In fact, when comparing things a patient can do to improve their health, the only thing ranking higher than adding regular exercise is to stop smoking if they are a smoker. Be advised, however, that this is a habit, and will be replaced by another habit. If you replace smoking with food, you'll gain weight. If it's going for a walk, you'll improve your health. If it's squeezing a ball, I guess you'll have a nice grip. This sure beats lung cancer, heart disease, reflux disease, and smoker's halitosis.

Depression and anxiety

When we are faced with stress, it triggers the fight or flight response. This may be helpful if you're being attacked by a wild animal, but it can present problems in social interactions. Treatment of anxiety and depression consists of three areas—medication, counseling, and exercise.

Depression and anxiety affect *serotonin, norepinephrine,* and other chemicals in the brain. Most of today's antidepressants work on serotonin receptors, with or without additional effect on norepinephrine receptors. These medications aren't necessarily more effective than older medications, but are generally considered to be safer. It is possible for them to actually worsen depression in some patients, so early follow-up is in order when starting or adjusting dosage of these medications.

You may not be able to change what is causing your symptoms, but you may be able to improve how you're processing it. That's where counseling comes in. The insight gained from counseling may also be effective at preventing a recurrence of symptoms.

Exercise does a lot of physical good, but it is also vitally important to mental health. Stress stimulates our fight-or-flight response. In the absence of doing something physical, this response is turned inward, where it does harm. Doing something physical puts this energy into a beneficial channel, where anxiety is released and chemical changes from exercise create feelings of well-being.

Your Health

Stress in general can also affect our digestive systems. Many of the same receptors that are affected by stress in our brains also exist in our guts. There's a good reason for this. Take the example of the python. A python is most vulnerable just after it has eaten a big meal. While it is resting and digesting, it can't shift energy very well to get away. If a python feels threatened soon after ingesting a huge meal, it will regurgitate the meal to facilitate an escape. Face it. A snake with a forty-pound calf in its gut just isn't going anywhere fast.

We're not wired all that differently than the python. If you've just downed a box of candy your mother sent you in a care package in college, and then a bear decides he wants some of your leftovers, you might just feel the urge to return to sender. (Defecating down the leg of your trousers in such a situation wouldn't be unheard of either.) In either case, your body is rapidly shifting from "rest and digest mode" to "fight or flight mode."

Heart Health

Hypertension

Blood is carried throughout your body from your heart via a high-pressure system called arteries. It is returned to your heart via a low-pressure system called veins. Your *systolic* blood pressure (top number) is the pressure at which your pulse can first be heard when your blood pressure is checked. Your *diastolic* blood pressure (bottom number) is the lowest number at which it can be heard. Systole is when your heart is contracting, creating the highest (systolic) pressure. Diastole is when your heart is relaxing and filling with blood between beats, creating the lower (diastolic) blood pressure.

The ideal values for healthy blood pressure are < 140 systolic / < 90 diastolic (< 130/ < 80 for a diabetic), and are based on studies of tens of thousands of people. People with blood pressures lower than these numbers had fewer heart attacks and strokes and generally lived healthier and longer lives than those with numbers above these values.

There are a number of factors that can affect blood pressure. Again, genetics play a role. If your mom, dad, grandparents, aunts, and uncles have high blood pressure, your risk of developing high blood pressure are higher than if they don't. Diet also plays a role, as a diet high in salt and meats and low in fruits and vegetables can also raise blood pressure. Some people are considered "salt-sensitive," meaning that high salt intake will significantly affect blood pressure. Smoking also plays a major role. Blood pressures can remain significantly elevated for up to two hours after exposure to smoke. There are twenty-four hours in a day so if you smoke even half a pack per day or are around someone who does, your blood pressure doesn't stand a chance.

So why is high blood pressure damaging? We've all seen a water hose with a leak in it. The higher you turn up the pressure, the more water shoots out of it and the bigger the mud hole gets. Imagine what's happening to the wall on the inside of that hose. Your blood pressure is a similar scenario. Over time, high blood pressure damages the walls of your arteries. Add to this *atherosclerotic* buildup of cholesterol plaques, which narrow the artery, and your demand for oxygenated blood quickly exceeds your supply.

Receptors in places like your kidneys send messages that supply is low, and they trigger your heart to pump harder and faster to get blood to your organs. Your heart gets the message from your kidneys: "I'm not getting enough blood. Some wild animal must have attacked me, and I must be bleeding. Constrict blood vessels to limit blood loss and pump harder to get blood to me." The end result is increased pressure and increased work on your heart. Over time, your heart will actually enlarge to accommodate the increased workload.

There are a number of blood pressure medications that work to overcome this pathway. Diuretics decrease volume so less blood is available to increase pressure. ACE inhibitors like Lisinopril block a pathway that causes constriction of blood vessels. Beta blockers work on receptors on the heart, causing your heart to not work as hard. Calcium channel blockers help to relax arteries and lessen constriction. Other medications work in other ways, some on the brain, to bring down pressure.

Thiazide diuretics and ACE inhibitors are generally considered first-line in the defense against high blood pressure because they have the best data to indicate that they prevent heart attacks and strokes and help patients live longer. We want to bring blood pressure down to a normal level, but that is simply a means to an end. Our ultimate goal with blood pressure medications is not simply the reduction in blood pressure, but the reduction in heart attacks and strokes. It's for this reason that we have a priority of which medications we like to use first.

With all this being said, remember that medications are only part of the treatment plan. Meeting goals like exercising for forty-five minutes five days per week can significantly reduce high blood pressure and, more importantly, reduce risk of cardiovascular disease.

Peripheral artery disease (PAD)

Just like you have blood vessels supplying your heart, brain, and genitals with blood, you have them supplying your arms and legs with blood as well. PAD can, like erectile dysfunction, be an early warning sign of heart disease.

The most common symptoms is something called *claudication*. Claudication is a crampy pain that you get, usually in your calves, when walking, especially uphill. The pain is caused by demand for blood that exceeds supply in narrowed arteries. This is analogous to angina (chest pain) associated with heart disease. Claudication generally improves with rest (since demand decreases and supply becomes sufficient). The degree of PAD can be measured by how far you can walk without having to stop.

If you complain of claudication, or PAD, your doctor may want to obtain something called an ankle-brachial index or ABI. This compares blood pressure in your ankle to your upper arm. A diminished ABI ratio indicates PAD.

If disease has progressed enough, you may need to see a vascular surgeon and have an arterial bypass to supply adequate blood to your feet. Many cases, however, can be effectively treated with exercise. This has been well-studied. Simply walking until the pain starts is not sufficient. Patients who manage to avoid surgery for PAD actually pushed beyond the pain, walking until the pain was bad enough to force them to stop.

One patient of mine in particular was exercising for thirty minutes a day five days per week, but he still had PAD. I recommended increasing his exercise time to forty-five minutes a day five days per week, and his vascular surgeon agreed. After just one month of the increase in exercise, his symptoms had dramatically improved and he managed to avoid surgery. It should be noted that if you are experiencing claudication, you should see your doctor. As this can be an early warning sign of heart disease, you may need to have further testing to be sure it is safe to start an exercise program.

Cholesterol

This issue is one of both nature and nurture. Excluding cultures that eat brains, you likely get roughly 75 percent of your cholesterol from what your liver produces and the other 25 percent from your diet. (Brains may contain up to ten times more cholesterol than eggs.) If you become a vegetarian, you may lower your cholesterol by up to 25 percent, but if you inherited the traits for very high cholesterol, this act alone may not be sufficient to get your numbers to target.

Your cholesterol should be low, right? What about good cholesterol versus bad cholesterol? What is a cholesterol ratio? First, understand that we all need cholesterol. Every cell membrane in our bodies is made of cholesterol. Cholesterol is also the building block to other hormones, including testosterone and estrogen. There are different types of cholesterol, but unless you're a molecular biologist, a book just on this isn't really necessary. Let's keep it simple and focused on what you need to know for your health.

Your body's total cholesterol the nutritional fact most often focused on, is actually not that important. What is more important is your ratio of high-density *lipoprotein,* or HDL (good) cholesterol to non-HDL (bad) cholesterol. The most well-known of these is the low-density lipoprotein, or LDL. In general, a high number here is bad for your health. There are much, much more complicated tests for further sub-analysis, but for our purposes, take a look at the triglyceride number. If this number is high (generally > 150), it is likely that a higher percentage of LDL particles are of a more artery-damaging subtype, and your numbers are worse than your ratio alone would suggest. If this number is low (generally < 150), it is likely that a lower percentage of the LDL particles are the more harmful subtype, and your numbers are a bit better than they at first appear.

Regular exercise, particularly first thing in the morning, can help to raise your HDL cholesterol, as well as lower your LDL cholesterol. If medication is necessary, statin medications, or HMG co-A reductase inhibitors, as they are properly known, are generally considered the drugs of choice. These medications work by inhibiting the slowest step in cholesterol synthesis in our livers. That's why baseline and regular blood tests are necessary while on these medications, as a potential side effect is liver toxicity.

The most common side effect of these medications is actually muscle aches, however. It is likely that the reason this occurs is depletion of co-enzyme Q10, which is involved in energy production in our bodies. It would likely benefit any patient who is on a statin medication to also be on a co-enzyme Q10 supplement. This supplement is readily available over-the-counter. I've had a number of patients who didn't tolerate a statin, but after starting a daily co-enzyme Q10 regimen and taking it while on the statin, they were able to tolerate it just fine without the muscle aches.

Please keep in mind, however, that statin medications can rarely cause more severe side effects. If muscle aches persist even with the addition of co-enzyme Q10, you need to see your doctor.

Another medication that can substantially improve your cholesterol is niacin, or vitamin B3. This vitamin is particularly good at raising HDL cholesterol. The most common side effect is flushing. This can be avoided most of the time by either taking the extended-release version or by taking an 81mg baby aspirin thirty minutes before the niacin. The dose of niacin necessary to achieve these cholesterol results is much higher than the typical daily intake (usually at least 500mg) so a supplement is generally necessary for this.

There are other classes of medications that may improve your cholesterol, but they are not considered the best for prevention of disease to our blood vessels. This is because our goal in treating cholesterol is not to improve your cholesterol profile; it is to reduce plaque build-up and ultimately reduce rates of heart attack and stroke. That's right. You would think that if you reduced bad cholesterol and raised good cholesterol, this would mean that your risk of heart attack or stroke would also decrease. Sadly, this is not always the case. Ideally, these numbers correlate, but it can take years to get the data necessary to show what a medication does beyond its numbers. That's why the newest, latest, greatest medication may not really be the best for you. Statins and niacin are considered the best because of their history of documented reductions in cardiovascular risk beyond cholesterol profiles.

Sleep, Obstructive Sleep Apnea, and Asthma

Insomnia

Most people will suffer from difficulty sleeping at some point in their lives. Insomnia can be a serious health problem and should not be ignored. Changes in routine, lack of environmental stimulus, especially sunlight, and stress can all adversely impact our sleep.

The first step in evaluating and treating insomnia is examining sleep hygiene. Sleep hygiene refers to your habits in the bedroom. Having a regular bedtime, not eating, reading, or watching television in the bedroom, and limiting excessive noise are all part of good sleep hygiene. A quiet room is usually best, but some patients will sleep better with a fan or sound machine to provide background or "white" noise.

A good sleep history will help your physician to accurately assess your insomnia. In particular, the spouse will often give key information, such as snoring, episodes of breathing cessation, sleepwalking, or periodic leg movements. Stress, depression, and anxiety can also seriously impact sleep. If you have good sleep hygiene, lack the symptoms listed above, and have had stress, depression, or anxiety addressed, sleep medication may be appropriate.

In treating insomnia with medication, it is best to go with the safest treatment first. Melatonin is the hormone your body secretes to cause you to sleep. You can obtain this over-the counter. You can also try 5-HTP, which is a precursor of melatonin and essentially does the same thing. Tylenol PM, which contains Benadryl, is also an over-the-counter option.

If these are ineffective, Trazodone is another option. It can cause some daytime sleepiness, as can many sleeping pills, but is generally considered safer for longer-term use than some of the other medications. One potential side effect of note with this medication is a risk of *priapism,* a prolonged, painful erection. This is rare, but requires prompt medical treatment if it occurs.

Other medications consist of many types of *benzodiazepines.* These medications work by increasing the frequency of chloride channels opening in neurotransmitters. Benzodiazepines can be habit-forming and should be used with caution. Long-term use should be avoided if possible.

Another sleeping medication that has garnered a lot of press is Ambien. This medication is pretty effective for short-term use, but some patients have been known to eat, sleepwalk, and do other activities while on this medication with no recollection of the events the next day. If you're already a known sleepwalker, tell your doctor before starting this medication, just to be on the safe side. It is also not generally recommended for long-term use.

If you do have a history of sleepwalking, periodic leg movements or restless leg syndrome, significant snoring, sleep apnea, or don't respond as anticipated to sleep medications, a sleep study is indicated. During a sleep study, you will be observed for these issues, and a specific treatment may be initiated to treat your specific symptoms.

Obstructive sleep apnea

Obstructive sleep apnea is a silent (or not-so-silent, if you ask a spouse) killer. Basically what is happening is that redundant tissue (i.e. floppy tissue in your throat, large tonsils, or just excessive fat around your neck) blocks your airway when you fall asleep. A partial blockage causes snoring, but occasionally the blockage completely blocks the airway and breathing ceases. When this happens, your tissues, including your heart, are starved for oxygen. After a few seconds, this triggers us to partially wake up—not enough to remember it, but just enough to start breathing again. Untreated obstructive sleep apnea can contribute to weight gain, excessive daytime sleepiness, increased risk of automobile or work-related accidents, heart disease, and death.

Most patients come to me for this at the request of their sleep partner. Contributing factors include obesity, neck circumference greater than seventeen inches, large tonsils or floppy soft palate, or nasal turbinate enlargement. Seasonal allergies, smoking, or second-hand smoke exposure may also worsen this disease.

If obstructive sleep apnea is suspected, you should have your doctor conduct a sleep study on you to determine the severity of your disease. You may be fitted for a machine providing continuous positive airway pressure (CPAP) or Bi-PAP (pressure varies with inspiration and expiration). This pressure essentially keeps redundant tissue in the throat from closing periodically and causing airway obstruction during sleep.

If weight is an issue, obstructive sleep apnea can often be cured or greatly improved with weight loss of as little as twenty pounds. If nasal or sinus disease is a contributing factor, treatment of this may significantly help symptoms.

The bottom line is that if you are having problems with sleep, you should see your doctor. It may be more serious than you think.

Asthma

Millions of Americans suffer from asthma. The coughing, wheezing, and shortness of breath can come on quite suddenly and can be debilitating. Asthma can be *intrinsic*, meaning that the symptoms occur without an obvious external stimulus, or *extrinsic*, meaning that the symptoms are triggered by an obvious stimulus.

Perfume, dust, seasonal or perennial allergies, a viral or bacterial respiratory tract infection, or cigarette smoke can all trigger an asthma attack. Avoidance of triggers is important when possible. Sometimes formal allergy testing is necessary when the triggers are not clear.

During an asthma attack, two main physiologic events are occurring—inflammation and a bronchospasm. Smooth muscle in the bronchi, triggered by intrinsic or extrinsic factors, constrict, causing the narrowing, reduced airflow, and characteristic wheezing sounds.

Albuterol is a beta agonist, meaning that it attaches to beta receptors on the smooth muscle of the bronchi, causing relaxation, and opening the airway. This can be given either with a couple of puffs through a metered-dose inhaler or through a nebulizer treatment.

Because the effects of the albuterol are short-acting, it gives only temporary relief. To treat the other cause of the airway narrowing and to provide definitive relief, an anti-inflammatory medication such as Prednisone is often required. Corticosteroid anti-inflammatory medications such as Prednisone can have systemic side effects, such as increased blood sugar, thinning bones, and contribution to cataract formation with chronic use, but if adequate ventilation of the lungs doesn't occur, none of this really matters. For short-term use (typically less than two weeks), the incidence of side effects is generally low.

Digestion

Gastroesophageal reflux disease (heartburn)

The esophagus runs just behind the heart in the chest. When hydrochloric acid from the stomach refluxes up the esophagus, it can give the sensation that your heart is on fire, hence the name "heartburn." There is a small muscle called the *gastroesophageal constrictor* that cinches off the opening of the stomach. Weakness of this muscle, overloading the stomach with large meals, or lying down soon after a meal can all contribute to the occurrence of reflux.

Carrying excess body weight can also add increased abdominal pressure, pushing acid upward. Smoking, excessive alcohol consumption, and excessive amounts of caffeine can also make this problem worse. Sometimes the upper portion of the stomach may herniate through the diaphragm into the chest, a condition called a *hiatal hernia*. This can also contribute to heartburn symptoms.

If you experience GERD, or heartburn symptoms including burning sensation, sour taste in your mouth, or chronic dry cough, there are some things you can do at home to treat it. If you are carrying excess body weight, even a ten to twenty pound loss can greatly reduce symptoms. If you're a smoker, stop. Limit caffeine and alcohol consumption. Eat smaller, more frequent meals, and avoid eating at least two hours before bedtime.

If symptoms persist despite these efforts, it's time to see your doctor. He or she may check you for bacteria called *Helicobacter pylori,* which can cause stomach upset. If this test is positive, a combination of antibiotics can cure the problem close to 90 percent of the time. If the test is negative, you may be started on a proton pump inhibitor (PPI) like Omeprazole. This medication works by turning off proton pumps, the acid producers of our stomachs. They are most effective when taken on an empty stomach thirty minutes before breakfast. You'll need to take these on a daily basis. Within twelve weeks, you should feel noticeably better.

If after twelve weeks symptoms have resolved, it may be reasonable to try going off the medication. This may be enough to allow your esophagus to heal, and some adjustments of your eating habits may be enough to keep a recurrence of symptoms away. Some people will need to be on these medications long term. If this is the case, your doctor should check you for vitamin B12 deficiency. There is an inherent need for our bodies to absorb vitamin B12 from our diets. An acidic environment is necessary for the intrinsic factor to be produced, so taking antacids may inhibit this along with the acid. Stomach acid is also a line of defense against bacterial infections from ingested food, so reducing acid may also impair your immune defense.

If you've had no improvement in your symptoms after twelve weeks of treatment with a PPI, it may be time to see a specialist like a gastroenterologist or general surgeon. An upper endoscopy procedure called and *esophagogastroduodenoscopy*, or EGD, as it is commonly known, will allow direct visualization of your upper digestive tract. Ulcers, hiatal hernias, or other diseases may be discovered with this procedure and more specific treatment plans developed.

Irritable bowel syndrome, or IBS

If you can't eat at certain restaurants without knowing in advance where the nearest bathroom is located, you may be an IBS sufferer. IBS can be either constipation or diarrhea-predominant. The intestines have a unique network of nerves around them, making abdominal pain different from most other types. When it stretches, we feel it. The pain can be intense. That's the way God makes us to let us know when it's time to take care of business. Gas, constipation, and diarrhea have sent numerous people to the emergency room.

Normal bowel motion is a process called *peristalsis*. When functioning properly, it's a smooth cascade. When this cascade gets out of sync, it can be terribly painful and distressing. Antispasmodic medications can be quite effective. Over-the-counter gas relievers can also be beneficial. Staying hydrated and getting plenty of fiber in the diet is also essential to healthy peristalsis.

Colon cancer, Crohn's disease, ulcerative colitis

Current guidelines recommend screening for colon cancer beginning at age fifty for those without a family history of colon cancer or polyps. Most people don't look forward to a colonoscopy. It's kind of like caving, except you're the cave. It does carry a risk of bowel perforation, which is a big deal if it happens. So why do it?

Most colon cancers don't start out as cancers, but

rather as pre-cancerous polyps that take a few years to turn cancerous. If these are found with a colonoscopy and removed, they never get the chance to become cancer. The chances of dying of colon cancer are much greater than dying from a perforation from a colonoscopy so getting screened is the way to go. Some patients refuse to have a colonoscopy for any reason. If this is you, I recommend at least doing an annual fecal occult blood test, as the first symptom of colon cancer is usually microscopic blood in the stool.

If you have a family history of colon cancer, Crohn's disease, or ulcerative colitis, beginning regular screening before you are fifty years old may be recommended. These diseases put you at greater risk for cancer, so talk to your doctor about them.

You should also talk to your doctor if you have rectal bleeding. By far, the most common cause of rectal bleeding is hemorrhoids, which is usually treatable without surgery. Sometimes the bleeding is caused by something other than hemorrhoids. If this is the case, the sooner you get it checked out, the better your chances of a good outcome.

Celiac disease

This disorder has gained a lot of attention recently. For some reason, some of us have an allergy to gluten. Untreated, this disease can cause IBS-type symptoms at first. As the body is repeatedly exposed to gluten, the inflammation gets worse and worse. Eventually, it may even increase risk of cancers.

The treatment involves eliminating gluten from the diet. The problem is that gluten is in so many processed foods.

Your Health

Successfully treating this requires you to do your homework and become somewhat of an expert on the subject.

This condition can be confirmed with bowel biopsy or blood tests. Predisposition to developing this disease can now also be determined with genetic testing.

Allergy/Immunology

Allergic rhinitis

Congestion, runny nose, sinus pressure, sneezing. Our *nasal mucosa* is the first line of defense for our respiratory tracts. Bacteria, viruses, allergens, or irritants will all stimulate increased blood flow, congestion, and increased mucus to some extent. Some patients suffer more in the spring, some in the fall. Some have symptoms lasting year-round.

The most effective thing you can do is to wash the area around your eyes, nose, and mouth with soap and water as soon as possible if you've been exposed to an infection, allergen, or irritant. Of the medication options, a corticosteroid nasal spray is the most effective when used correctly.

These sprays work most effectively when used daily during the allergy season. Systemic effects of the corticosteroid is generally considered to be too low to cause long-term problems. The technique of spraying them is also important. If you spray it straight up, it tends to just drip out. Sinuses in the nose run horizontally, so tilting your head forward and spraying back into the nostril tends to deliver the spray more effectively.

Nasal and oral antihistamines can also be used

in conjunction with the corticosteroid nasal sprays. If you're doing all of the above and your symptoms are still uncontrolled, it may be time to see an allergist. An allergist can test you for specific allergens and may initiate immunotherapy (allergy shots) as part of your treatment to relieve symptoms.

Sinusitis

The most common complaint I see in medicine is sinusitis. The majority of sinus infections are caused by viral infections. Viral infections still cause fever, sinus pain, congestion, and drainage, but antibiotics don't help them. Taking antibiotics for a viral infection only gives you side effects, most commonly diarrhea. Demanding antibiotics for a viral infection may give you diarrhea in addition to your original illness.

Bacterial sinus infections typically last greater than seven to ten days, affect one side more than the other, and often were preceded by a viral infection. Smokers or those with allergic rhinitis may be more susceptible to secondary bacterial infections due to more underlying congestion, causing difficulty in getting sinuses to drain.

Most acute sinus infections can be treated with a narrow-spectrum antibiotic, such as amoxicillin. Using a broader spectrum antibiotic increases your risk of side effects and may reduce the coverage of these medications with continued overuse. If you've been on an antibiotic recently or there is suspicion that you have a resistant strain of bacteria, a broader-spectrum antibiotic may be necessary.

It is very important to take your antibiotic as prescribed and to finish your prescription to prevent development of resistant strains of bacteria. Never take anyone else's

Your Health

prescription, share your prescription with others, or save some for later.

Medication is only part of the treatment for a sinus infection. A sinus massage can help facilitate drainage. If your sinuses won't drain, the infection may linger. Have you ever noticed that after a sneeze your sinuses seem to open up for a few seconds? This is caused by a sympathetic response of the *trigeminal nerve*. There are three branches of this nerve, exiting the skull just above the eyes, over the cheeks, and over the chin. Gently massaging these areas can simulate the benefits of a sneeze without the mess of a sneeze.

Skin

Skin cancers

Probably the best and worst types of cancers a person can get are both skin cancers. Melanomas are bad news. They are usually pigmented and may be flat or raised. Excessive sun exposure can increase the risk of developing melanomas. Australians have much higher rates of this type of skin cancer due to their fair complexions and intense sun exposure.

It is important to know the A–B–C–Ds of pigmented skin lesions. A is for asymmetry. If you cut a lesion in half with an imaginary line, it should look roughly the same on both sides. This is symmetry. An asymmetrical lesion should get your attention. B is for border. A border should be smooth and sharp. Beware of jagged or ragged edges. C is for color. A very dark, multi-colored skin lesion, or a lesion which is changing color should be evaluated. D is for diameter. If a skin lesion is enlarging, especially rapidly, get it checked out. Knowing your A–B–C–Ds could save your life.

Basal cell carcinomas rarely spread elsewhere, but can be locally invasive. They may have a waxy appearance with a rolled border. These can usually be removed in the primary care setting, but sometimes the location of these lesions may make seeing a specialist necessary. For lesions on the nose, an ear, or face in general, seeing a plastic surgeon or a dermatologist with special training in a procedure called *Moh's* may be necessary.

There are many other types of skin cancers, but the better-known ones are melanomas and basal cells, and squamous cell carcinomas. Squamous cell carcinomas often start as pre-cancerous lesions called *actinic keratoses,* but in contrast to these will often be thicker.

Pre-cancerous lesions

Actinic keratoses (AKs) are red areas of the skin often with white, flaky areas superficially. These can be difficult to differentiate from irritated dry skin in the winter time. Untreated, they may progress into squamous cell carcinomas. AKs can be destroyed with liquid nitrogen. If they are extensive, they may be treated with a destructive cream. This is ideally done in winter or when sun exposure can be limited, as it will be quite irritating and often requires a "rescue" corticosteroid cream after completion of treatment with the destructive cream to relieve skin irritation.

If there is a question as to the identity of a skin lesion, it's usually better to have it biopsied than frozen, as freezing may distort or destroy key identifiers and incompletely treat the condition.

Rashes and eczema

Rashes can be caused by fungal infections, allergic reactions, irritants, or autoimmune phenomena. Many times, the rash is self-limited and goes away before a definitive diagnosis can be made. Important factors to discuss with your doctor include if it itches, where it started, exposures, and what you've done to treat it already. Some conditions, such as psoriasis, may have a genetic component.

Eczema tends to be worse in the winter and can have many variants. *Keratosis pilaris* is an eczema variant commonly seen on the back of the upper arms in winter months with raised red bumps. It can be effectively treated with a prescription lotion or cream. *Dishydrosis* or *pomphylox* involves the hands and can be very difficult to treat.

A basic rule of dermatology is that if it's wet, dry it, and if it's dry, wet it. An ointment is a wet gooey base. A lotion dries more quickly. A cream is somewhere in between.

Take a cool rather than hot shower, apply a cream rather than lotion, and use topical corticosteroid preparations intermittently; all of the above can effectively treat eczema in most cases.

In general, a rash or other skin condition is something very difficult to diagnose or treat over the telephone. If it's bad enough to require treatment, it's bad enough to see your doctor sooner rather than later.

Hair loss

People seem to want what they can't have. Those with curly hair want straight hair. Those with straight hair want curls. Those who are bald would take either. A number of conditions can cause hair loss—fungal infections, autoimmune disorders, and heredity. The timing, distribution, and severity of the hair loss can be important clues to both diagnosis and treatment.

Telogen effluvium refers to loss of a percentage of hair diffusely. The average hair grows for two years, and then goes dormant for three months. At any given time, many hairs are in the growth phase while others are dormant. Sometimes hair can "sync" their phases. Pregnancy is a common example of this phenomena. A pregnant woman's hair gets very thick as hair follicles sync to the growth phase. After delivery, a high percentage may go into dormancy and hair falls out at an alarming rate. This corrects itself over a few months.

Male pattern baldness is a sex-influenced trait, meaning that the genes for this are located on both the X and Y chromosomes. In men, it is a dominant trait under the influence of high levels of testosterone. In women, who have lower testosterone levels, it is recessive. If women have two copies for male-pattern baldness, however, they can experience baldness.

There are two main treatments for hair loss. One involves increasing blood flow to the scalp. Topical formulations of Minoxidil like Rogaine dilate blood vessels, increasing blood supply to atrophied follicles. These preparations are successful for a number of patients.

Another treatment involves inhibition of the conversion of testosterone to *dihydrotestosterone,* a more potent form. The medication Propecia is the same medication as Proscar, used for enlarged prostate, but only 20 percent of the dose.

Endocrine

Diabetes

Your pancreas has both endocrine and exocrine functions. Exocrine function refers to the enzymes released into your intestine to break down fatty foods. Endocrine function refers to substances released into your blood that work primarily on blood sugar. Parts of your pancreas called *Islets of Langerhans* produce these substances. Your have alpha cells and beta cells in the Islets of Langerhans.

The substance released from alpha cells is called *glucagon*. Glucagon pulls sugar into your blood to mobilize it for energy. A form of this substance is used in medicine to reverse overdose of diabetes medications or beta blockers (used for the heart).

Insulin is produced in beta cells. Diabetes mellitus is a disease that affects these cells. In type one, there is destruction of these cells from some reaction, thought to be autoimmune, where the body attacks itself. The exact cause of this is unknown, although theories exist. People who suffer from type one diabetes mellitus require injections of insulin to process carbohydrates in their diet because the cells that produce it in their pancreas have been destroyed.

People with type one diabetes mellitus are usually young when they develop the disease and tend to be thin.

Type two diabetes mellitus, which is much more common, usually presents in adulthood, but is now being seen in adolescence and even childhood. It is caused by insulin resistance, meaning that your body produces insulin, but it is less effective at pulling sugar into your cells for use.

Whether a person has type one or type two diabetes, persistently elevated levels of blood sugar causes damage to blood vessels. This damage increases a person's chances of heart attack, stroke, blindness, kidney disease and failure, and impotence via damage to blood vessels supplying these organs. It can also cause a loss of sensation to limbs (diabetic peripheral neuropathy), which can in turn lead to amputations. Most of the horror stories people hear about diabetes are related to poor control of the disease.

There are both hereditary and environmental factors contributing to development of diabetes. Some lucky people can eat whatever they want, never exercise, and be significantly overweight, yet not develop diabetes. Don't get me wrong; their lifestyle is still in and of itself a hazard to their health. They're just genetically lucky regarding this disease. Others will develop diabetes despite maintaining a normal body weight, regular exercise, and a low glycemic index diet.

It is still important for you to do all these things, however, if you are susceptible to developing diabetes, as this may prolong the amount of time you have before requiring medications to treat it, the amount of time before requiring insulin, and it may significantly reduce your risk of the complications of diabetes listed above. I assure you that you are not wasting your time in investing in a healthy lifestyle.

Your Health

Risk factors for developing diabetes include family history, being overweight or obese, leading an inactive lifestyle, and poor diet. Warning signs that you may be developing diabetes or that your diabetes may not be controlled include excessive thirst, hunger, or urination. You may also have some unintentional weight loss as your body is no longer able to make use of all the carbohydrates you're eating. You may develop a patch of darkening skin around your neck that looks like dirt. This is called *acanthosis nigricans* and can be a sign that you're developing diabetes. If you're having any of these symptoms, you should consult your doctor to discuss them.

The cornerstone of treatment for type two diabetes mellitus is lifestyle modification. Success begins and ends here. Meeting a target of forty-five minutes of exercise five days per week dramatically improves outcomes. Insulin is necessary to break down carbohydrates, but not proteins or fats. In the days before medications, your best bet for controlling diabetes likely would've been a low-carb diet similar to the Atkins or South Beach diet of today. It is important to get some carbohydrates in your diet, as these are your major sources of fiber and antioxidants, but these should be low glycemic index foods.

Foods with a low glycemic index take your body longer to break down. They tend to have a lot of fiber and are found mostly in fresh fruits and vegetables. Refined foods tend to have a higher glycemic index. Low glycemic index foods help you maintain better control of your blood sugar, as the rise in blood sugar is more gradual and the drop in response to insulin is less precipitous. It is thought that this rapid drop in blood sugar seen with high glycemic index foods is a stimulus for overeating. The same effect is not generally seen with low glycemic index foods.

For those of you who have diabetes, let me leave you with this word of encouragement: It's not all your fault. The natural course of the disease is a progressive decline in pancreatic function. If you're having increasing difficulty in managing your blood sugar despite doing the things listed above, that doesn't mean you've failed. It doesn't mean you're less of a competent patient. It simply means that you need some adjustment in your game plan. Diabetes medications and even insulin are sometimes necessary as part of the plan.

Fatigue

"I'm just so tired," is a common complaint we hear in primary care. By far, the most common cause is just de-conditioning. Over time, a sedentary body loses muscle mass, strength, ability to regulate heat, and works less efficiently. Work on lifestyle modification, including addition of regular exercise and a healthy diet can to some extent reverse this.

Other causes of fatigue commonly include anemia, hypothyroidism, and depression. Rarely, adrenal insufficiency, testosterone deficiency in men, menopause in women, or vitamin deficiency can also be involved. In fact, vitamin D and B–12 deficiency isn't all that uncommon, and both are easily correctible. Chronic obstructive pulmonary disease is an often-missed contributing factor. Checking a chest X-ray and pulmonary function test, especially in a current or former smoker, can be important.

Neurology

Headaches

There are many types of headaches. Tension, migraine, cluster, and sinus are just a few. Regardless of the particular type of headache, there is often a tension component. The major muscles of the neck include the trapezius, located over the back of the neck and upper part of the back, and the scalene and sternocleidomastoids, located laterally. Treating tension of these muscles can significantly improve symptoms.

For migraine headaches, triptans like Imitrex or Maxalt are good treatment for stopping a headache that has already started in some patients. Migraines are vascular headaches, and triptans work by constricting blood vessels. These medications may be contraindicated in some patients and are available by prescription only. Medication types used to prevent migraines include beta blockers (also used to control blood pressure), antidepressants, and anti-seizure medications.

Riboflavin, a B vitamin, may play a role in migraine prevention as well. Riboflavin is water soluble, so our bodies don't readily store it. If you get too much, you'll likely get rid of the excess in your urine. Anyone who has taken a B vitamin has likely noticed the bright yellow urine when the excess is eliminated. Taking a daily B vitamin is a safe and often effective way to help prevent migraine headaches.

Co-enzyme Q–10 is another over-the-counter supplement that has benefit in migraine prevention for many patients. Taking 100mg three times daily may cut incidence by as much as half.

For new, changing, worsening headaches, or headaches without a clear cause, you should see your doctor. A headaches diary, in which you rate your headache on a scale such as 0 (no headache) to 5 (emergency room) morning, afternoon, and night for one month will often help your doctor in diagnosing and treating your headaches.

Seizures/epilepsy

Every winter at least one child gets a high fever and experiences a seizure. A febrile seizure, though a traumatic experience, conveys no increased risk of epilepsy later in life. There can be a genetic predisposition to epilepsy, and seizure activity can manifest as generalized convulsions, a focal repetitive activity, or just "zoning out."

If seizure activity is suspected, brain imaging like an MRI and a consultation with a neurologist is warranted. A person experiencing a seizure should not drive until cleared to do so by a licensed neurologist. A number of treatments are now available, and the majority of seizure disorders can be well controlled.

Restless leg syndrome

Restless legs can severely impair the ability to get a good night's sleep. Simple dehydration is the most common cause of these muscle spasms. Making sure to stay adequately hydrated is a good place to start treatment for this condition. If symptoms persist or worsen, see your doctor.

A number of things can contribute to restless legs. Electrolyte imbalance, too much or too little iron, or vitamin deficiency are important factors and should be checked with blood work. A sleep study or nerve conduction study may also be warranted. The same medications used to treat Parkinson's disease at a lower dose are often beneficial for restless leg syndrome.

Parkinson's disease

Parkinson's disease is a progressive neurological disorder often first noticed by a tremor of one hand with the appearance that the person is rolling a pill—hence the term "pill-rolling tremor." It can cause a hunched posture, a shuffling gait with short, slow steps, and a loss of expressiveness of the face.

Those with a family history of Parkinson's disease may be at increased risk of developing it themselves. There are a number of medication treatments for Parkinson's disease, each with their benefits and potential risks. One over-the-counter supplement that may have some benefit in slowing the progression of the disease is co-enzyme Q10. Doses of up to 2,400mg per day have been studied in use with Parkinson's. This is much higher than the typical dose of 300mg daily for migraine headache prevention. If you suffer from Parkinson's disease, ask your neurologist about the role of co-enzyme Q10 in your treatment.

Men's Health

Erectile dysfunction

Viagra was originally developed as a heart drug. Its use in erectile dysfunction came from an interesting side effect that it was noted to have. (Not all side effects are bad.) It works by dilating blood vessels. This is important to understand because most (not all) cases of erectile dysfunction are vascular problems. Hypertension, diabetes, obesity, poor diet, and lack of exercise can all contribute to erectile dysfunction.

This goes back to the supply and demand point from hypertension. If you have blood vessels that are narrowed by atherosclerotic plaques, arterial wall thickening from hypertension or diabetes, or just plain lack of exercise, less blood gets to your genitals, contributing to a weaker, smaller erection.

The good news is that our bodies can adjust. If we challenge our bodies with exercise in a controlled environment, over time our vasculature will improve. Subsequently, supply will improve and you can expect a stronger, fuller erection.

Be cautious about ED pills, preparations, and "natural" male enhancements on television or the Internet. Some of these can be dangerous because of exacerbating effects on hypertension, and many just won't work. They might offer a money-back guarantee, but who is really going to want their money back badly enough to admit their insufficiencies to get it? I'd recommend discussing ED treatments with your doctor before purchasing any.

Another important consideration with erectile dysfunction is that it can be an early warning sign for heart disease. Erectile dysfunction can precede heart disease by as much as five years.

Urinary tract health

"The male curse," as it's sometimes known; an enlarged prostate can impair the ability of a man to pass urine from his bladder. Symptoms of an enlarged prostate can include frequent urination, having to get up many times at night to urinate, a weak stream, stopping and starting, and erectile dysfunction. These symptoms can also occur with prostate cancer so you should see your doctor if you are experiencing these.

There are two main types of medications used to treat an enlarged prostate. Alpha blockers dilate the part of the urethra that passes through the prostate, allowing urine to pass more freely. These medications start working fairly quickly, but have a side effect of *orthostatic hypotension, a sudden drop in blood pressure related to a change in body position*, especially when starting the medication or increasing the dose. Rising slowly when starting or increasing the dose can help prevent you from hitting the floor when you go to answer the door.

The other type is a medication that inhibits the conversion of testosterone to its more potent form, *dihydrotestosterone*.

This medication takes longer to show benefits, but can be used along with an alpha blocker and may actually shrink the prostate over time. This medication may have the side effect of reducing sexual performance and should not be handled by women who are nursing, pregnant, or may become pregnant, as it may cause problems with the sexual development of male infants or fetuses.

The over-the-counter supplement saw palmetto may offer some benefit to prostate health. Lycopene, which is found in tomatoes and watermelon, is also excellent for prostate health and health in general.

Women's Health

Infertility

Infertility in women can result from a number of causes including infection, lack of ovulation, obstruction of the reproductive tract, or chromosomal abnormalities. Gonorrhea and chlamydia can cause pelvic inflammatory disease, increasing the odds of a tubal pregnancy or lack of conception.

Polycystic ovarian syndrome can cause irregular menstrual periods and irregular hormone levels, causing an inability to ovulate. Treating PCOS can help to regulate menstrual cycles and increase odds of ovulation. If an obstruction of the reproductive tract is suspected, a procedure called a *hysterosalpingogram* may be done to evaluate patency of the tract.

Chromosomal abnormalities and advanced maternal age are also issues to infertility. Anyone with recurrent miscarriages should be evaluated for a chromosomal abnormality. As many women put off having a family to focus on a career, they may be passing the window of opportunity to reproduce. Beyond age thirty-five, menstrual cycles become less regular and odds of successful, uncomplicated pregnancies greatly decrease.

There are new technologies available for fertility, including in-vitro fertilization, embryo adoption, and surrogacy. The technology now exists to choose many features of your child, including the sex. However, along with this ability comes a greater responsibility to hold true to your ethical values in planning your family.

Urinary Tract Health

The most common predisposing factor to getting urinary tract infections is simply being female. A shorter urinary tract makes for getting infections more easily. Cranberry juice may reduce *E. coli*'s ability to adhere to the urinary tract so drinking it regularly may reduce the recurrence of *E. coli* urinary tract infections. Once you have an infection, however, cranberry juice isn't likely to cure it.

Staying hydrated, urinating frequently, urinating after intercourse, and wiping front-to-back are all good habits to reduce chances of infection. Often a woman will come in with a urinary tract infection after traveling due to not drinking enough water and going too long without urinating.

Bone density

Thin women, white or Asian women, and elderly women are all at increased risk of thinning of the bones. Adequate dietary calcium and vitamin D are important, but probably the most-neglected preventative measure is regular weight-bearing exercise. You don't have to be a power lifter to benefit from strength training.

Strength training builds both muscle and bone, reducing not only risk of fracture from a fall, but also risk of falling in the first place. Have you ever noticed that frail, elderly women often seem to have difficulty staying warm? Muscle, among other benefits, keeps us warm.

To keep your bones healthy, get regular weight-bearing exercise. Drink mild or dairy products. Get some sunlight (in moderation). Realistically, you should probably get 1,000 units of vitamin D3 in the summer and closer to 2,000 units daily in the winter months. This is a bit higher than the recommended daily allowances commonly given.

Medical Genetics: The Future of Medicine

Nature versus nurture

Twenty years from now, I expect medical genetics to play a very large role in how we apply treatments. Right now, you can order a test online, spit in a cup, and in two months know where your ancestors likely originated, what your health risk for various diseases are compared to the average person, and how you would likely respond to a number of medications.

The biggest risk with this information is theft of potentially damaging information, making it difficult or expensive to get life or health insurance. The benefits, however, are tremendous. If you knew you were at great risk of colon cancer or diabetes, would it change your health habits? Would it change what your physician recommended as screening guidelines?

The technology also opens up an ethical dilemma. If we can know, should we? Much of the information out there is preliminary and has the potential to cause undue worry. If you knew you were a carrier for a potentially dangerous disease, would it affect your decision to have children? Would your spouse also want to be checked? Would you want to take advantage of specialized in-vitro techniques with pre-implantation diagnostics?

Expected drug response

There is a tremendous amount of variation in how different people respond to the same medication. In one person, a medication may be broken down quickly, requiring multiple doses per day. In another, the effects may last more than one day. In yet another, the same medication may cause liver toxicity.

In this area, I think it is desirable to pursue a study of genetic response. This can save lives. Why suffer an adverse effect when it can be avoided? I expect this to be part of mainstream medicine within a couple of decades.

Traits

Here we step onto a slippery slope. If you knew you were extremely likely to go bald, you might invest early in medication to slow the process before all your hair fell out. If you knew you were genetically more likely to be a distance runner than a sprinter, you may go into cross country running rather than the 200 meter. Still, even traits are influenced not only by nature but also by nurture, and the jury is still out on just how many genes influence each of these traits.

Labeling even ourselves can be dangerous, and it is important to remember that genetics is only the beginning. If we are to be ethically responsible with ourselves, we should be even more so with our children. The goal is to be proactive with this information; nothing more and nothing less.

Faith

Not everything in health care can be easily explained. Sometimes, despite valiant efforts, people die. Other times, people make unexpected recoveries we can only classify as miraculous. No matter how much you work to stay healthy and no matter how skilled your health care team, only God decides when and how you will die. I've seen a few miracles of my own, and here I share a few of them to inspire you and to give God due glory.

In March 2004, while on a two-week international elective in medical school, two of our physician team members, Matt and David, became seriously ill. They had contracted gastroenteritis—nausea, vomiting, and diarrhea. It may not sound like much here, but consider this: you can work with a cough or runny nose. You can't very well work with your rear end leaking like a sieve. Remember also that we were in a third world country, not the United States. Gastroenteritis is actually a common cause of death in third world countries.

Having come to help others, Matt and David now found themselves helplessly on the other end of health care. Our trip was with an international group called Word of Life Ministries. While physicians, nurses, physician's assistants, dentists, and students ministered to patient's health needs, Word of Life Staff ministered to their spiritual needs. Now they lay dehydrated, weak, and lethargic in their bunk beds.

In their time of need, Matt and David made a request that surprised some. "Pray for us," they asked. "We teach others to trust in God for their needs. Who is better able than God to heal us?" We prayed, and within thirty minutes, it was as if they had never been ill. Here they were, physicians, knowing full well what their best options were to get well; knowing that gastroenteritis takes days if not weeks to recover from fully; and they knew exactly where to go for help.

You may make the argument that they had a quick-acting type of gastroenteritis that only lasted a few hours. As a physician, I can tell you that it is not at all medically likely to either stop so quickly or to get re-hydrate, re-energize, and regain appetite so quickly. As a physician, I can tell you that this was a legitimate miracle. God healed them!

A couple of years later, now as a resident, I had seen a lot of suffering and pain working in the hospital. Depressed by what I was seeing on a daily basis, I prayed one night for God to let me see a patient survive from an event that so many times they do not. Not long after that, a patient came into the hospital in cardiac arrest. Despite repeated efforts, repeated shocks, she was not responding.

Figuring there was nothing to lose by letting a resident take a turn in the resuscitation efforts, they let me have a turn. I used the defibrillator paddles for the first time, and surprisingly her heart continued beating afterward. She was then taken to the intensive care unit with the expectation that at least her family would have time to say goodbye. Knowing what kind of condition she was in, I went home that night with a heavy heart.

Your Health

When I arrived at the hospital to make rounds the next morning, I was surprised to see her family in the ICU waiting room. "Oh, no!" I thought. "I've kept her alive only to have her become a vegetable!" I was at the bottom of an emotional well. Why would God let this happen? Why, when I prayed to see someone survive, would he allow *this* to happen? Why would he do this to me? To her? To her family?

When I made rounds, I heard that she had moved and responded to questions. Later that day, she was taken off the tube that had been placed down her throat to breath for her and she was talking. Within two more days, she was walking, talking, and even dancing in her hospital room. One of her sons, who had been out of the country, was able to make it to see her. She only lost one thing through the whole ordeal … her pain.

Her family reported that she had been in chronic pain and was always complaining about it. Since her near-death experience, she had had no pain at all. She felt great; in fact, the best she had ever felt. None of us had ever seen a recovery like this. She stayed in the hospital for about one week. Having lived a long and full life, her family elected against life-saving procedures should her heart stop again, making her "do not resuscitate," or DNR, status. The night before she was to go home, her heart stopped again. This time she died, but not before she got to say goodbye to her family and experience the happiest days of her life pain-free.

A few years later, now working in a local medical group, I had settled in to a comfortable routine that was interrupted one cold January morning with the news that a close friend of mine had been in a serious car accident. Details were limited at the time, but what was known was that they were air lifting him to the hospital. This couldn't be good. As a physician, I knew that anyone airlifted from an accident has a very high likelihood of dying.

I fell to my knees and immediately started praying through the tears. My partners at work moved my patients to their schedules and prayed with me before I left for the hospital to see my friend. In my heart I feared the worst, but knowing his family would be there at the hospital, I had to be strong.

I later found out that he had hit a patch of black ice and rolled his SUV. He had been wearing his seatbelt, but the force of the impact from the roof collapsing as the SUV rolled was so strong that it had partially ejected him, and the SUV then rolled on top of him.

He was on a desolate stretch of road, so it was a while before anyone came upon him. In fact, his work had called his home. Reaching his wife, they asked her if he was coming into work that day. She was panic-stricken. He had left an hour ago!

When first responders arrived on the scene, he was only lucid enough to tell them his name and where he worked. They found a church directory in his car and called the church to find out where he lived and whom to contact. Soon police arrived at his house. He and his wife had two small children and were expecting number three. His parents had been visiting and inexplicably decided to stay another day. The Lord had provided childcare at this crucial moment before they even knew it was needed.

When I arrived at the hospital, I found probably twenty people from church in the waiting room. I had to filter any emotion I felt with each new piece of information, as I was now responsible for helping everyone understand what was going on with him medically. I was as scared as they were.

He looked worse than I had expected. He was so swollen that I wouldn't have known who he was had they not told me. As we were about to go home for the night, his wife had just come out from seeing him and reported that they had just placed him on something called *Levophed*. My heart sank. Levophed, or "leave 'em dead" as it was ominously nicknamed, was used as a last resort to keep blood pressure up enough when someone was about to die. I swallowed hard and kept a straight face as I told her good night.

I communicated with Rick Brooks, a staff member with Word of Life and good friend of mine and Matt's. Yes. This was the same Matt who had been sick in Central America a few years before. Rick was in Australia to set up the South Pacific Ministry, and I sent him a list of specific prayer requests: 1. For Matt to come off the Levophed. 2. For his pulse to come down to normal (He had lost a lot of blood, and the pulse rises in this situation.) 3. For his blood pressure to stabilize. 4. For him to come off the ventilator. As we went to bed in despair, not knowing if our friend would live or die, Rick called the board together and prayed for Matt. While it was night here, it was already the next day in Australia, and prayers went up on Matt's behalf around the clock.

The next morning I called Matt's nurse for an update. From her tone, I could sense surprise. She said that he was off the Levophed, his pulse was down, his blood pressure was up, and they were hoping to start weaning him off the ventilator later that day. When I saw him later that day, to my surprise, he looked better than the previous day.

The prayers continued, and one week after his near-fatal

crash he was out of the hospital. He broke several bones and had to have some rehabilitation, but he was back to work in three months time. This was a miracle.

Another miracle happened on a smaller scale, but is no less impressive. A new patient came to my practice, having recently relocated to pastor a local church. His name is Dr. Phil. Not that Dr. Phil, but Dr. Phil Martin. He one day noticed a lesion growing on his leg and came in to get it checked out. As it looked suspicious, we took a biopsy of the edge with something called a punch biopsy. It basically looks like a miniature biscuit cutter. This one was 4mm in diameter.

The pathology report came back positive for skin cancer. I called Phil and let him know that we'd need to do a complete excision to get rid of the whole cancer, as we had only biopsied an edge to see what the pathology report would show. He came back and we did a full excision. Before he left, he asked if we could pray, which we did. To my amazement, the pathology report showed no abnormal cells. What I expected was for it to say "clear margins." This is surprising, as the whole lesion was much larger than 4mm and we only biopsied one small edge. There was obviously more cancerous tissue, but where did it go? I know the spot was correct, as I left the original sutures from the punch biopsy intact when I excised it with the full lesion.

So if the site was correct, how did it disappear? Could the biopsy have stimulated his immune system to fight off the cancer? Not likely. Could the diagnosis be wrong? Well, it was biopsy-proven! I have to give credit where it's due. As I told Phil, God healed his leg. I just cut out a chunk of it. This too was a miracle. Amazing? Yes. Surprising? Surprisingly not. I'm skeptical by nature, but I pray for wisdom and skill in caring for the patients God entrusts to my care. I can't say that it's completely surprising when He heals them, as I've come to appreciate that He can. It never stops being amazing, however, that He does.

I hope you've found this book helpful and empowering to you. Remember that your life is a gift from God. Be proactive and enjoy it!